*Major Problems in Obstetrics and Gynecology*

A series of monographs designed to explore in depth specific problems in these related disciplines, and to offer reviews of the most complete and up-to-date information available on topics in the study of human reproduction and of the female reproductive system.

Other monographs scheduled for publication in this Series:

Hogan and Fink: *Hematologic Problems in Pregnancy*
Bieniarz: *Angiography and Placental Localization*
Glicksman: *Radiotherapy of Gynecological Malignancy*

*With Contributions by*

JULIUS H. BOLGLA, M.D.
Formerly Director,
Department of Anesthesia

MARTIN B. KASS, M.D.
Resident in Obstetrics and Gynecology

MARSHALL BENNETT TAYLOR, M.D.
Resident in Obstetrics and Gynecology

*All of Michael Reese Hospital and Medical Center, Chicago, Illinois*

A set of 50 color slides duplicating the photographs in Chapter 17 is also available from the publisher.

# LAPAROSCOPY, CULDOSCOPY AND GYNECOGRAPHY

*Technique and Atlas*

MELVIN R. COHEN, M.D.

Senior Attending Physician, Department of Obstetrics and Gynecology, Michael Reese Hospital and Medical Center; Associate Professor of Obstetrics and Gynecology, Chicago Medical School; Director, The Fertility Institute, Chicago, Illinois

VOLUME 1 IN THE SERIES

MAJOR PROBLEMS IN OBSTETRICS AND GYNECOLOGY

EMANUEL A. FRIEDMAN, M.D.
*Consulting Editor*

W. B. Saunders Company  Philadelphia • London • Toronto

W. B. Saunders Company: West Washington Square
Philadelphia, Pa. 19105

12 Dyott Street
London, WC1A 1DB

1835 Yonge Street
Toronto 7, Ontario

Laparoscopy, Culdoscopy and Gynecography: Technique and Atlas

SBN 0-7216-2650-5



Print No.: 9 8 7 6 5 4 3 2

*Dedicated to My Patients—*
*Fertile and Infertile—*
*and Especially to Those with Obscure Pelvic Pathology.*

# Foreword

With this first volume in the series Major Problems in Obstetrics and Gynecology, we feel that we have begun to fill a great void, for detailed, comprehensive sources of information in encyclopedic or monographic form are not otherwise available in our specialty to students, house officers, generalists, and specialists. Our textbooks tend to be superficial in pertinent areas of great interest, and our specialty journals are frequently inundated with trivia. Under the auspices of the W. B. Saunders Company, we have embarked on a long-term project to try to correct these deficiencies. Eminently qualified authors have been sought out for this task, so as to provide scholarly and practical dissertations comprising readily usable information and summarizing clinical aspects of diagnosis and treatment of the major problems we will be presenting.

This first volume deals quite appropriately with techniques which afford the clinician diagnostic tools unparalleled in gynecology. The rebirth of gynecologic laparoscopy and its burgeoning popularity are undoubtedly the result of recent refinements in technique and, more pertinently, in instrumentation, specifically the introduction of cold light fiber optic technology. The simplicity of laparoscopy and its relative advantages over culdoscopy, here treated in a critical and balanced manner, account in large measure for both its growing acceptance and its rapidly expanding scope of applicability. Visual clarity, panoramic view, and potential for limited surgical exercises are additional attractive features.

Dr. Melvin R. Cohen, long active in the research and practical aspects of infertility and widely recognized for his expertise in culdoscopy and gynecography, writes with considerable authority based on extensive experience in the performance and modification of laparoscopic observation and surgery. This book is a distillate of his experience, and it reflects his tempered judgment, keen perception, and articulate literary style. The book treats primarily the practical aspects of the techniques, stressing pertinent features of anesthesia, indications, contraindications, and complications. The use of photography for appropriate documentation is detailed as well. The work provides the degree of thoroughness expected of Doctor Cohen. Of special note is the final chapter which contains an atlas of wonderfully detailed photographs illustrating a spectrum of pathologic conditions observed during culdoscopy and laparoscopy. These pictures illustrate the wide range of application of these techniques to many of the major problems in obstetrics and gynecology that this series will undertake to elucidate in due course.

EMANUEL A. FRIEDMAN, M.D., MED. SC.D.

*Boston*

# Preface

My interest in laparoscopy was initiated by a visit to the Broca Hospital and Clinic in Paris in 1966. There Raoul Palmer graciously invited me to observe "gynecologic celioscopy," as he calls this technique, performed especially in the infertile woman. I was impressed with the magnificent view of the pelvic organs and with how easily such ancillary surgical procedures as tubal dilatation, biopsy, and cautery were performed. Later I was privileged to observe Patrick Steptoe, at Oldham Hospital in England, perform interval tubal sterilization via laparoscopy. Despite my earlier enthusiasm for culdoscopy, I realized that the abdominal approach had certain diagnostic, surgical, and photographic advantages.

As background, a historical review of laparoscopy (also called peritoneoscopy or celioscopy) is presented in Chapter 2. Due credit is given to the great innovators Ott, Kelling, Jacobaeus, and others who brought to the gynecologist this invaluable technique of viewing the pelvic organs with lighted instruments.

The modus operandi of laparoscopy is illustrated and the actual technique is described in detail. The various instruments that can be used are too numerous to describe, but the discussion includes all that are readily available to the American gynecologist.

The safe introduction of carbon dioxide gas into the peritoneal cavity is also discussed in detail. This is one of the most important steps in laparoscopy, and most of the complications that have been reported are due to faulty technique at this stage. My teacher and former associate Irving F. Stein, Sr., M.D., was an enthusiast of pneumoperitoneum. Used alone or combined with hysterosalpingography (gynecography), this is a valuable technique in the diagnosis of obscure pelvic disease (Chapter 16). My experience with pneumoperitoneum was a decided advantage in laparoscopy.

Indications and contraindications of both laparoscopy and culdoscopy are discussed, and complications are reviewed in detail. A description of ancillary procedures, such as lysis of adhesions, biopsy, cyst aspiration, and tubal sterilization, is presented as well.

Photography is important for documentation of findings and for teaching, and a black-and-white atlas of gynecologic endoscopy has therefore been included. A supplementary atlas of the original Ektachrome slides from which these illustrations were made is available from the publisher. Some of these slides will have been seen previously: at the American Fertility Society meeting in April, 1967, I presented an exhibit entitled "Culdoscopy versus Peritoneoscopy" that included a collection of Ektachrome transparencies illustrating the potential of endoscopy and especially laparoscopy. S. Leon Israel, M.D., editor of *Obstetrics and Gynecology*, encouraged me to write an article on the subject, and this was published with color plates (Cohen, 1968*a*).

Also in 1968, two motion pictures were produced: "Peritoneoscopy: Technique and Cinematography" and "Tubal Sterilization via Peritoneoscopy." The latter was made with the assistance of Alan Silverman, M.D., senior resident at Michael Reese Hospital and Medical Center, and both films are available on loan from La Rue Films, Inc., of Chicago. In 1969 our two residents, Marshall Bennett Taylor, M.D., and Martin B. Kass, M.D., with my cooperation, produced a third motion picture, "Operative Laparoscopy: Tubal Sterilization," which was shown at the meeting of the Chicago Gynecological Society on May 16, 1969. At that time the paper that appears as Chapter 9 of this book was presented.

For some time I had been exploring the possibility of avoiding the use of general anesthesia in laparoscopy. With the cooperation of the Department of Anesthesia of Michael Reese Hospital, and the former director of that department, Julius H. Bolgla, M.D., I am now performing laparoscopy under local anesthesia plus Innovar (Chapter 4). A new motion picture, "Laparoscopy: Refinements in Technique and Anesthesia," soon to be available, demonstrates this procedure under neuroleptanalgesia.

Joseph Rovinsky, M.D., of Mount Sinai Hospital, New York, requested that I rewrite the chapter on peritoneoscopy for Davis's *Gynecology and Obstetrics*, originally prepared by Ruddock in 1939. In doing so I felt the need to amplify this material and present it as a book with atlas, and this was the origin of the present work. I feel privileged to have been invited by Emanuel A. Friedman, M.D., of the Harvard Medical School and Beth Israel Hospital, to present my material in monograph form for this new Saunders series. As our former chairman, Dr. Friedman had given me every assistance in the establishment of laparoscopy at Michael Reese Hospital. I trust that in writing this book I will stimulate interest in endoscopy and provide additional teaching material for meaningful courses in both laparoscopy and culdoscopy.

I wish also to honor my good friend Albert Decker, M.D., the "father of culdoscopy." It is my hope that despite the current enthusiasm for laparoscopy, culdoscopy will continue to be taught and performed at medical centers. The two techniques complement each other, and they are compared in Chapter 13.

I have been nearly overwhelmed with requests to teach laparoscopy. Therefore, this text has been prepared to give a step-by-step detailed description of the technique. I have tried to make the procedure as simple as possible and to show how to avoid problems in anesthesia, in the introduction of the pneumoperitoneum, and finally in the introduction of the trochar and laparoscope. It is strongly suggested that one person, or, preferably, a small team of gynecologic endoscopists, be trained at each large hospital and medical center so that this invaluable technique will be available to the entire staff. Although laparoscopy, known since the early part of this century, has been discarded and then rediscovered at intervals, I am confident that with the availability of fine optical instruments and safe anesthesia the technique is here to stay.

MELVIN R. COHEN, M.D.

*Chicago*

# Acknowledgments

Grateful acknowledgment is due the operating room staff of Michael Reese Hospital for their invaluable help in establishing laparoscopy, first as an experimental technique and now as a routine diagnostic and operative procedure. I want to apologize to my colleagues for any inconvenience caused by my taking additional operating room time for laparoscopic photography.

I have been fortunate to have had the cooperation of L. Streifeneder and L. Wetterman of the Eder Instrument Company, who supplied me with fine instruments and encouragement. Mr. Streifeneder even came into the hospital operating room to insure that the laparoscopy instruments and camera attachments were in perfect order.

The endoscopic photographs are my own. The other illustrations are the work of Gunter Deutch, La Rue Films, Inc., June Hill Pedigo, medical illustrator, and Stanley Kaval and Obie Evans, photographers.

For their patience in typing the many drafts of the manuscript, Mrs. Jeanne Lieberman and my wife Miriam deserve my appreciation.

Our present department chairman, Antonio Scommegna, M.D., and our esteemed senior obstetrician and gynecologist at Michael Reese Hospital, J. P. Greenhill, M.D., were kind enough to review my material.

The interest and enthusiasm shown by the staff of the W. B. Saunders Company have greatly stimulated my efforts.

Finally, I wish to acknowledge the understanding and enthusiasm of my children, Nancy and Alan. And most helpful, most encouraging, and the most important of all was my wife, Miriam.

MELVIN R. COHEN, M.D.

# Contents

*Chapter One*

# INTRODUCTION. MODUS OPERANDI OF LAPAROSCOPY

Laparoscopy (peritoneoscopy, celioscopy) is endoscopic visualization of the peritoneal cavity through the anterior abdominal wall after establishment of a pneumoperitoneum. Unlike culdoscopy (transvaginal endoscopy), this technique is also useful to the internist and surgeon evaluating abdominal problems, especially liver disease. Gynecologic laparoscopy refers to the application of this technique for the diagnosis of obscure pelvic diseases.

It has been said that the gynecologist must have eyes at the ends of his fingers so that he can delineate the size, shape, and position of the uterus and evaluate the adnexa. Pathologic conditions due to cysts, inflammation, or endometriosis must be differentiated from the normal tube and ovary. The vaginal or bimanual examination requires training and experience, and even the trained gynecologist frequently has difficulties making a diagnosis. Symptoms such as severe pelvic pain are sometimes unexplained by what can be palpated vaginally. The need for refinements in diagnostic techniques is obvious.

Inspection of the external genitalia, the vagina and cervix, as well as palpation and percussion of the abdomen, are very important and when combined with bimanual examination lead to the correct diagnosis in the majority of patients. When the diagnosis is in doubt, the gynecologist needs to take a good look at the internal genitalia. If this can be done without laparotomy, safely and under minimal anesthesia and discomfort, it would appear to be a worthwhile proce-

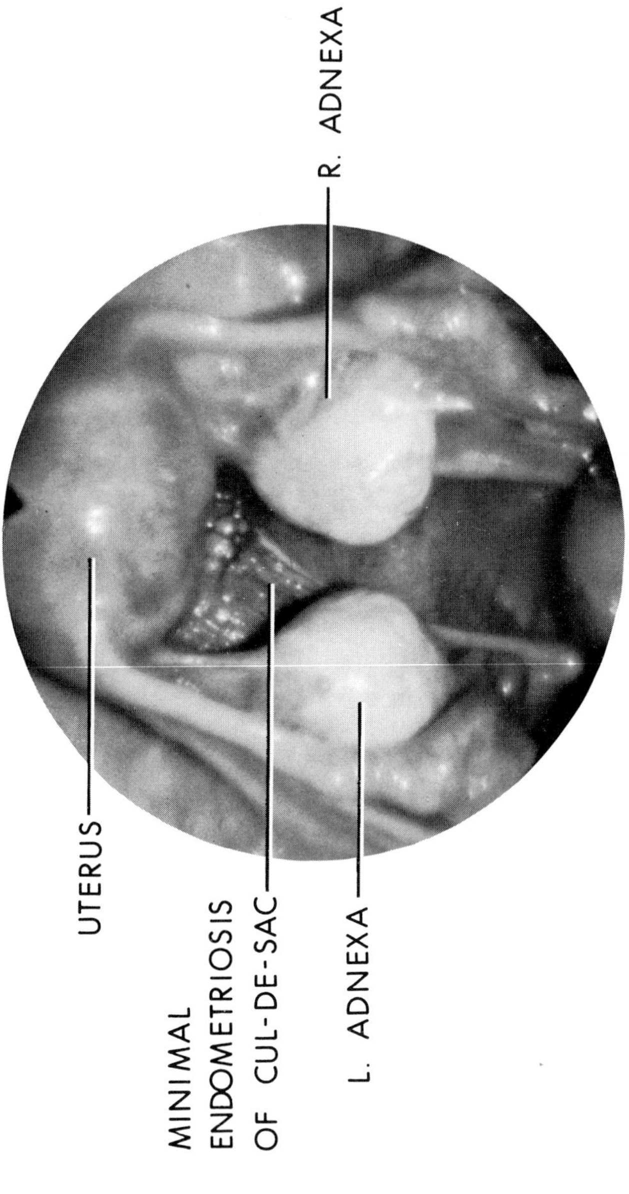


*Figure 1–1.* Panoramic view at laparoscopy of normal uterus and adnexa with minimal cul-de-sac endometriosis. (From an Ektachrome transparency.)

dure. By means of laparoscopy the gynecologist can obtain the same view of the pelvic organs (Fig. 1–1) as is seen at laparotomy

Although this method has been known since 1901, Palmer in 1947 perfected the technique of "gynecologic celioscopy" by showing that the pelvic organs could be better visualized with the use of an intra-uterine patency cannula. The uterus and its appendages can be moved freely up and down using the cannula as a lever.

## MODUS OPERANDI

Figure 1–2 is a schematic drawing of gynecologic laparoscopy. A pneumoperitoneum is performed so that the intestines are separated from the pelvic organs. The bladder is catheterized. A uterine patency cannula is inserted through the cervix and hooked into position. This serves as a lever so that the uterus and its appendages may be moved up out of the cul-de-sac to enable the surgeon to observe structures behind these organs. The cannula may also be used for tubal patency, employing either methylene blue or indigo carmine dye for injection. The patient is placed in Trendelenburg

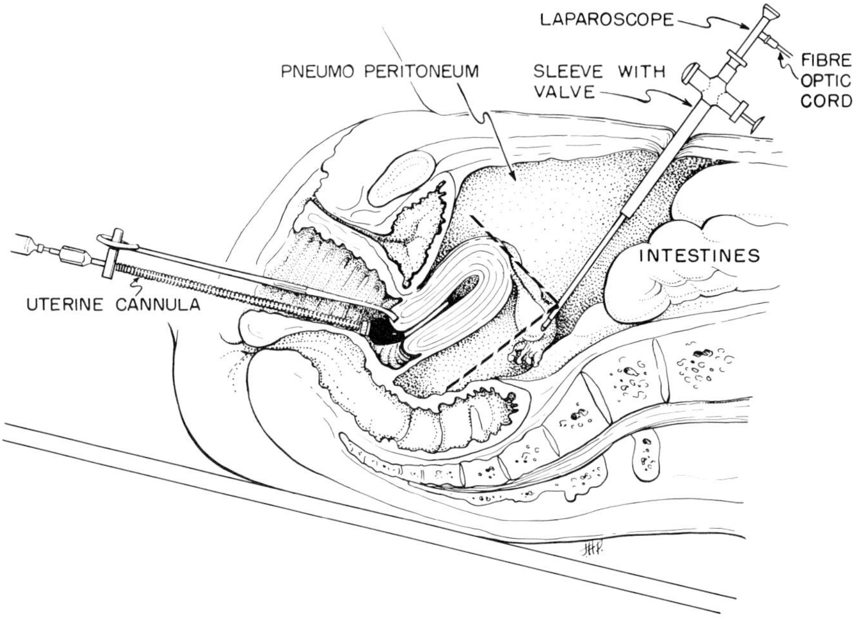


*Figure 1–2.* Schematic drawing of gynecologic laparoscopy. (From Cohen, M. R. [1968*a*]: Culdoscopy vs. peritoneoscopy. Obstet. Gynec. *31*:310.)

position to facilitate displacement of the intestines out of the pelvis. The laparoscope passes through the trochar sleeve, which is fitted with a valve to prevent the escape of gas from the peritoneal cavity. A light cord from the power supply is attached to the laparoscope.

### *The View Obtained at Laparoscopy*

Those who have never seen this technique performed are usually amazed at the panorama of the pelvic and lower abdominal organs. The view obtained at laparoscopy is identical to the appearance of these organs at the time of laparotomy and serves to immediately orient the gynecologist. On the other hand, the internist, who is more concerned with upper abdominal problems, might be confused by the appearance of a small ovarian cyst or an endometrial implant. One must have a thorough knowledge of gross anatomy and gross pathology for the proper interpretation of findings.

The peritoneum over the previously catheterized bladder may be seen, and the round ligaments are clearly visualized. Should the uterus be in retroflexion, it can be moved anteriorly with the patency cannula so that the cul-de-sac may be seen. The uterosacral ligaments are easily identified and pathologic aberrations of the cul-de-sac, such as endometriosis, are clearly definable.

The fallopian tubes may be identified from the uterine end to the fimbriated end, and the entire surface of both ovaries may be seen unless obscured by lesions. If it is not possible to see the underneath surface of the appendages, an additional instrument, such as a probe, may be inserted easily through the abdominal wall. With the probe, structures may be moved about and, if the instrument is graduated in centimeters, measured. In contradistinction to culdoscopy, a full panorama of the pelvic organs is immediately visualized at laparoscopy. It is then possible to advance the laparoscope further so that all details are clearly seen.

With the intra-uterine cannula, dilute indigo carmine or methylene blue dye may be injected to demonstrate tubal patency. The gynecologist should be able to differentiate between the gross appearance of the nonovulating ovary and one that clearly shows the effects of ovulation, viz, the corpus hemorrhagicum, corpus luteum in various stages of development (including the corpus luteum verum), old areas of luteinization, the graafian follicle and luteinized follicles. The time for the most dramatic visualization of the ovary is immediately after ovulation when the corpus hemorrhagicum may be seen. This structure usually occupies from one-half to one-third of the ovary and shows intense vascularization. The area of ovum escape may have the appearance of a stigma with or without coagulum. There may be evidence of recent hemorrhage. We have compared the appearance of the corpus hemorrhagicum to that of a bloodshot eye.

The size, shape, and position of the uterus may be easily evaluated via laparoscopy. Color of the organ varies with the intensity of illumination.

A uterus enlarged by an intramural leiomyoma must be differentiated from an early pregnancy. A pelvic examination that always precedes laparoscopy may help in making this distinction. The older literature describes the value of laparoscopy in diagnosing pelvic tuberculosis. This disease has become infrequent and I have not had any experience with this condition. The reddish or purplish implants compatible with the gross diagnosis of endometriosis frequently involve the peritoneum, uterosacral ligaments, cul-de-sac, and ovaries. Biopsy is usually unnecessary to confirm this diagnosis. Early malignant lesions of the ovaries may be diagnosed on gross inspection and biopsy. Ovarian carcinoma with metastases and ascites may also be diagnosed in this manner. It is my opinion that whenever curettage is indicated for bleeding states, endoscopic examination, either by culdoscopy or laparoscopy, is of value in determining possible ovarian etiology.

Although the gynecologist is able to visualize the upper abdomen, he is not qualified to evaluate the gross appearance of the liver, whether normal or abnormal. We have been frequently requested by the internist to perform upper abdominal laparoscopy to visualize the liver and gallbladder and to aid in obtaining liver biopsy. Upper abdominal laparoscopy is an entirely different procedure and should not be performed by the gynecologist. The gastroenterologist trained in gastroscopy will find this technique easy to learn and rewarding.

*Chapter Two*

# HISTORICAL BACKGROUND

Ott of Petrograd, in 1901, was the first to introduce optical inspection of the abdominal cavity. He placed his patients in extreme Trendelenburg position at a 45° angle on a special table with shoulder braces and supports for the legs. By means of culdotomy, vaginal retractors, and a head mirror with incandescent light, he was able to visualize the pelvic and abdominal organs. Ott was primarily a vaginal gynecologic surgeon and he demonstrated that pelvic and even intestinal surgery could be accomplished with this technique. He showed that in steep Trendelenburg position negative pressure occurred and the bowel was displaced out of the pelvis into the subdiaphragmatic space. Deep general anesthesia was further required to keep the visual field free from loops of intestines. His remarkable operation was called "ventroscopy."

Kelling of Dresden presented a paper in Hamburg in 1901 (published in 1902), entitled "Ueber Oesophagoskopie, Gastroskopie und Kölioskopie." The last-named procedure (celioscopy) was demonstrated on a dog, and this first-recorded method of abdominal endoscopy is quite similar to the technique now employed. A pneumoperitoneum was first produced with a needle and filtered air. A trochar was then inserted through an anesthetized area in the abdominal wall and a thin Nitze cystoscope inserted. In this way Kelling was able to visualize the contents of the abdominal cavity. Nitze had introduced the cystoscope in 1878; Kelling was the first to extend the use of this valuable instrument to view a body cavity by creation of an artificial opening.

Jacobaeus of Stockholm, in 1910, was the first to describe laparoscopy, as he called this technique, in the human. Jacobaeus was unaware of Kelling's earlier report, and the technique he employed was not as advanced as Kelling's. Jacobaeus did not use a preliminary pneumoperitoneum. He utilized the technique chiefly in patients with ascites—the ascitic fluid was removed and air substituted. He wrote numerous papers from 1910 until 1923 and published a monograph reporting 45 laparoscopic examinations of patients chiefly suffering from liver diseases.

There is a great deal of controversy as to whether Jacobaeus should be given credit for introducing laparoscopy or whether the credit should go instead to Kelling, the innovator of this technique, which he called "Kölioskopie." In a reply to Jacobaeus, published in 1910, Kelling stated that he had successfully performed Kölioskopie on two patients. He also stated that the method had been used frequently in the Veterinary Institute of Dresden during physiology experiments on dogs. He failed to publish any further reports until 1923. In an address before the German Surgical Society he stated that the post-World War I economic state in Germany compelled him to use this diagnostic method to avoid prolonged hospitalization and the expense of exploratory laparotomy. Kelling simplified his original method by piercing the abdominal wall only once with a beveled trochar, grooved to accommodate a small tube for transmission of air. He maintained that in the living patient the mobility of the intestines, receding from the slow thrust of the trochar, prevents bowel perforation. Kelling's simplified technique was a step backward; his original technique with preliminary pneumoperitoneum in the dog was far safer.

Bernheim, an American, in 1911 described a method of abdominal exploration by means of a proctoscope inserted through a short incision in the epigastrium. With illumination by an electric head light he was able to inspect the lesser and greater curvatures of the stomach, the gallbladder, and the liver. Bernheim further made an incision into the stomach to explore for gastric ulcer.

In 1912, Nordentoeft of Copenhagen, unaware of the previous work of Kelling and Jacobaeus, described an instrument called a trochar-endoscope. The instrument was useful in (1) suprapubic cystoscopy, (2) arthroscopy of the knee, and (3) physiologic experiments involving observation of the body cavities of animals. Nordentoeft utilized his instrument to view the pelvis of a female cadaver and obtained the first endoscopic photograph of the internal genitalia. He did not report any clinical experience with laparoscopy.

In 1912, Tedesko of Vienna reported his experience with a method of laparoscopy after Jacobaeus. He utilized this technique only on patients with ascites.

In France, papers by Renon (1913, 1914) and Rosenthal (1913) followed the work of Jacobaeus. Renon chiefly used this technique for diagnosing pathologic conditions of the liver. In Italy, Roccavilla

(1914, 1920) designed an instrument that permitted the source of light to remain outside the abdomen. His trochar tube also permitted the accommodation of a Nitze cystoscope. In Germany, Schmidt (1914) was pessimistic concerning his experience with laparoscopy. Johnsson (1916) of Finland reported his experience with both thoracoscopy and laparoscopy, relating the difficulties of interpretation of the endoscopic findings.

Orndoff of Chicago published a paper in 1920 entitled "The peritoneoscope in diagnosis of diseases of the abdomen." Since Orndoff was primarily a roentgenologist, he, unfortunately, published his paper in the Journal of Radiology. Consequently, his work did not gain recognition among gynecologists.

Orndoff invented his own instrument, which was a modification of a thoracoscope, and he devised a trochar that was ground with three faces, each with sharp, pointed margins to fit a cannula. The cannula was of Size #15 French to permit endoscopes to be inserted through it. An automatic valve was attached to the cannula to prevent the escape of gas. The instrument had an electric filament lamp and optic similar to the ordinary cystoscope. His technique is outlined in the following steps: (1) selecting the site, (2) preparing the field, (3) administering the local anesthesia, (4) producing a pneumoperitoneum, (5) conducting such x-ray examinations as were deemed necessary, (6) inserting the trochar and cannula of the peritoneoscope, (7) adjusting the amount of gas in the peritoneum to give the proper distention, (8) inserting the lamp and lens system and making observations with the aid of the x-ray and fluorescent screen, (9) monitoring the position of the patient to facilitate the observations in the screen and peritoneoscope, and, finally, (10) withdrawing the gas from the peritoneum and closing the wound at the site of puncture. Orndoff used oxygen for pneumoperitoneum and reported his technique in 42 cases, including cases of (1) tubercular peritonitis, (2) hemoperitoneum and hydroperitoneum, (3) extra-uterine pregnancy, (4) salpingitis, (5) ovarian cysts and tumors, (6) abdominal tumors, and (7) liver disease. He further utilized the technique of transillumination of the abdominal wall.

Korbsch, in 1921 and 1922, developed new instruments and also demonstrated the need for a pneumoperitoneum produced by a separate needle. Korbsch called his technique "Die Laparoskopie, nach Jacobaeus," but actually he improved Jacobaeus's technique and even utilized the pneumoperitoneum for abdominal x-ray examinations.

In 1924, Steiner, an American, described what he thought was a new discovery, "abdominoscopy." In Steiner's technique a stab wound was made through the skin, and a trochar and tube were inserted through the abdominal wall while the patient's abdominal muscles were contracted. Frequently, the puncture was made with the patient erect. After penetrating the peritoneal cavity, the trochar was removed and the abdominoscope, a modified cystoscope, was introduced. Filtered air was then pumped into the peritoneal cavity. It is remarkable that some 14 years after the Kelling and Jacobaeus reports, Steiner stated that "Abdominoscopy has never been performed on the living patient or on the cadaver," and that he was unable to find any papers dealing with the theoretical or experimental phases of the subject.

A paper entitled "Endoscopy of the abdomen: abdominoscopy," by Nadeau and Kampmeier of Chicago (1925), presented an extensive review of the literature. Despite the numerous reports up to this time, these authors stated that the method was seldom used. They said:

"After exploring with light and lens the open cavities of the body, such as the rectum, bladder, esophagus, trachea, and bronchi, the idea of making the closed cavities accessible to the eye became more insistent. The potential of such endoscopic exploration was too fascinating not to explore."

Zollikofer of Switzerland, in 1924, was chiefly concerned with laparoscopy in liver disease. He employed carbon dioxide for pneumoperitoneum because it is easily and quickly absorbed. In 1929, Kalk reported his experience with 100 laparoscopic examinations and described his own instrument. His system of lenses produced a foroblique (135°) viewing system and he used a pneumoperitoneum needle. Kalk's laparoscope, with certain modifications, is still used today.

Ruddock, an American, published his work in 1934 on "peritoneoscopy," as he called it, and stimulated interest in the United States. He perfected his own peritoneoscope, pneumoperitoneum needle, and trochar and trochar sleeve. He also described ancillary biopsy instruments. Ruddock's peritoneoscope was modified after the McCarthy cystoscope. He utilized air for the pneumoperitoneum, local anesthesia, and reported an initial series of 200 cases, which was later augmented to 2500 cases.

In 1937, Hope suggested the use of peritoneoscopy in the differential diagnosis of ectopic gestation. He reported 10 cases, several of which were from the service of Dr. Ruddock.

Other Americans influential in the development of laparoscopy included Anderson (1937), Benedict (1938), Meigs (1939), and Beling (1939). Anderson reported the use of this technique for tubal sterilization. Beling discussed the indications as well as the contraindications of peritoneoscopy, the term used by the American school. He stated:

"As the technique of peritoneoscopy has progressed, miracles have been expected of the instrument simply because the requesting physician was not thoroughly familiar with what it can and cannot do. The peritoneoscopist must not fail to realize this fact and to take the trouble to explain the indications. Only thus can he hope to put the instrument to the best and most widespread use, and only thus can he hope not to be called to perform peritoneoscopic examination on a patient with an appendiceal abscess or an intestinal obstruction. It is even more important that the peritoneoscopist preserve at all costs a critical attitude in selecting cases, and that he be not influenced by others to examine patients with the peritoneoscope when he has any doubts as to the existence of contraindications. Too often an instrument instead of its operator is condemned when it has been faultily or injudiciously used."

Beling was chiefly a gastroenterologist. He classified peritoneoscopy as a diagnostic procedure not in competition with exploratory laparotomy. He apparently was not too impressed with its value in the diagnosis of pelvic disease unless a large uterine fibroid or a large ovarian cyst floating freely in the peritoneal cavity on a long pedicle was present. He was impressed, however, with its value in the diagnosis of ectopic pregnancy.

Decker (1944) stated that he had used the peritoneoscope as an aid in the diagnosis of upper abdominal and pelvic disease. He found that the route to the pelvis by abdominal endoscopy, even with the aid of vaginal manipulation and various postures, did not give uniformly satisfactory results. He stated that failure of proper visualization was usually due to the presence of intestinal loops and the inability to isolate the pelvic organs properly. In an effort to improve the usefulness of the endoscope in pelvic diagnosis, he became interested in the vaginal route. He stated that in contradistinction to peritoneoscopy, culdoscopy gave uniformly good results and that when the procedure of culdoscopy is carried out in properly selected cases, one can obtain all the visual and some of the palpable information that is otherwise only obtained by laparotomy. He demonstrated that in the knee-chest position, puncture of the cul-de-sac created a spontaneous pneumoperitoneum. Thus, an endoscope could be safely inserted through the thin rectovaginal septum and the pelvic organs visualized. Decker insisted that this procedure must be performed under local anesthesia.

In 1946, Palmer perfected the technique of "gynecologic celioscopy." In 1947 he reported 250 cases in which this technique was used without any serious accident. He stressed the value of an intra-uterine patency cannula. Pneumoperitoneum was produced at the rate of 300 to 500 cc. of gas per minute. In his 1947 publication Palmer stated that the technique in the majority of his patients was performed under local anesthesia, although general anesthesia could be employed. He warned that the intra-abdominal pressure should not exceed 25 mm. of mercury. Palmer was familiar with culdoscopy, but he preferred celioscopy because there was less chance of pelvic infection and surgical techniques could be more easily applied.

Frangenheim, since 1957, has published many excellent treatises on laparoscopy. His personal experience included 1850 peritoneoscopies and culdoscopies performed without serious complications. In a paper, "Technical errors in peritoneoscopy," he discusses such complications as emphysema, air embolism, intestinal perforation, hemorrhage, burns from hot incandescent lamps, pulmonary and cardiac problems during anesthesia, and postoperative infections. He stated that infection is rare and is usually due to tubal insufflation or hydrotubation reactivating chronic or subacute pelvic infection, rather than to the peritoneoscopy itself.

Frangenheim stressed general anesthesia, extreme caution in inducing a pneumoperitoneum, and avoidance of puncture through a previous laparotomy scar. The laparoscope of Frangenheim is one of the standard optical instruments available today.

Clyman, in 1963, described "operative culdoscopy." In this technique culdoscopy is performed usually under local anesthesia. The puncture site is enlarged, creating a 3 to 4 cm. incision, and the cannula with the culdoscope is reinserted through the enlarged opening. Clyman not only cauterizes endometrial implants and adhesions, but he is able to perform ovarian and tubal surgery. Tubal ligation is feasible under local anesthesia. He states that patients may be discharged within 24 to 48 hours after the operation. Antibiotics are prescribed for all patients.

Clyman lists as contraindications dense adhesions involving the intestines or lateral pelvic wall in the vicinity of the iliac vessels or in patients with vaginal or pelvic infections. In his report in 1968, out of a group of 400 operative culdoscopies, 15 had complications. Six had reactivation of a chronic salpingitis, one patient with a wedge resection of the ovaries developed an ovarian abscess, and another patient, following wedge resection, developed fever and pelvic pain. After vaginal removal of an ectopic pregnancy, one patient developed a retroperitoneal abscess. Six additional patients had low grade fevers which resolved with antibiotics.

Excellent textbooks on laparoscopy are available in German (Frangenheim), French (Thoyer-Rozat), Italian (Albano and Cittadini), and English (Steptoe's "Laparoscopy in Gynaecology,"

1967). An additional exemplary text is Wittman's "Peritoneoscopy" (Budapest, 1966), which has been translated into many languages, including English. Decker recently brought out a new edition of his "Culdoscopy" in 1967. It is extremely comprehensive and beautifully illustrated, with many photographs in color.

In America two recent publications, one by Fear (1968) and another by Cohen (1968*a*), have stimulated great interest in laparoscopy, which is presently competing favorably with culdoscopy among American gynecologists. More recently, Siegler and Berenyi (1969) reported their experience in 114 patients, 44 of whom had permanent tubal sterilization. General anesthesia was used and no major complications occurred.

Inspection of the abdominal cavity and the pelvic organs by means of a lensed instrument is known by many different names. The following are examples: *Kölioskopie* (Kelling, 1902), *ventroscopy* (Ott, 1901), *Laparo-thorakoskopie* (Jacobaeus, 1910), *organoscopy* (Bernheim, 1911), *peritoneoscopy* (Orndoff, 1920), *abdominoscopy* (Steiner, 1924), *endoscopy of the abdomen: abdominoscopy* (Nadeau and Kampmeier, 1925), and *la coelioscopie gynécologique* (Palmer, 1947). The confusion in nomenclature is illustrated by Frangenheim, who refers to the technique as *Kölioskopie, coelioskopie, laparoscopy* and *peritoneoscopy* in various publications.

The instruments available to the American gynecologist are all termed "laparoscopes" and perhaps, for the sake of simplicity and uniformity, the technique should be known universally as "laparoscopy."

*Chapter Three*

# TECHNIQUE OF LAPAROSCOPY

Preoperatively the patient is given a cleansing enema the night before or the morning of surgery. Food and fluids are withheld for at least eight hours. Preoperative medication should include atropine, 0.4 mg., plus a narcotic such as meperidine, 75 to 100 mg. intramuscularly, approximately one hour prior to surgery. A standard operating room table is employed, and the patient placed in gynecologic (lithotomy) position with the legs and thighs somewhat extended to allow access to the abdominal wall.

Nonalcoholic solutions are utilized for skin sterilization since cautery may be employed as part of ancillary laparoscopy techniques. Our preference is a povidone iodine* solution, which is an adequate disinfectant and nonflammable

Anesthesia is begun, the bladder is catheterized, and a bimanual pelvic examination is performed. A patency cannula is inserted and clamped into place (Fig. 3–1). Any standard self-retaining patency cannula may be used. A dilute indigo carmine or methylene blue solution is prepared so that tubal patency studies may be performed if indicated. Should curettage or endometrial biopsy be necessary, it usually follows the completion of the endoscopic procedure. The abdomen need not be shaved except in the area near the umbilicus, but should a laparotomy be contemplated, the abdomen would be completely prepared. A pneumoperitoneum is performed (Fig. 3–2). As gas fills the peritoneal cavity (Fig. 3–3), percussion aids in deter-

---

*Betadine, The Purdue-Frederick Co., Yonkers, N.Y.

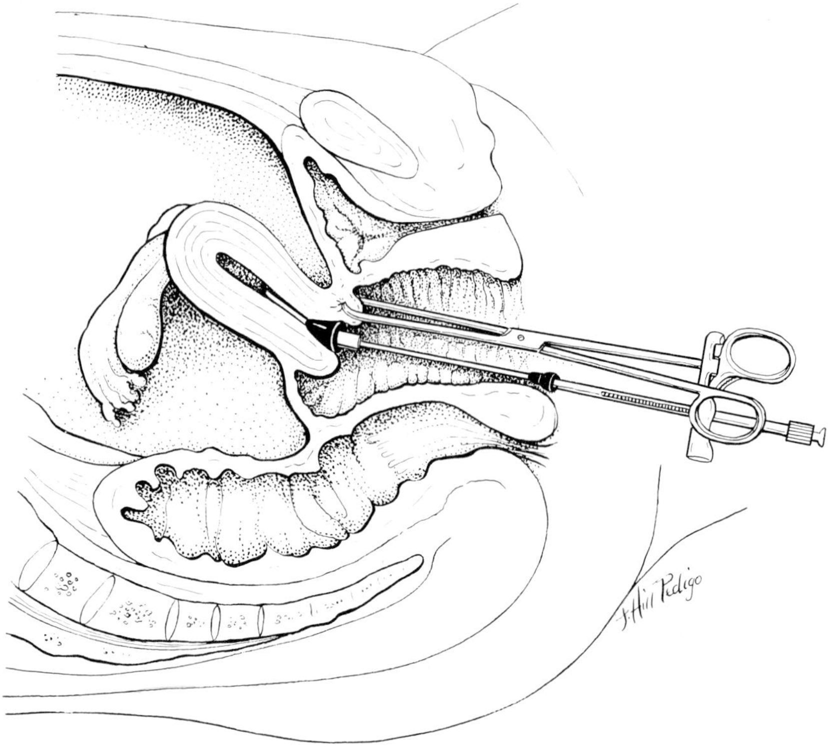

*Figure 3–1.* Uterine patency cannula in position (schematic).

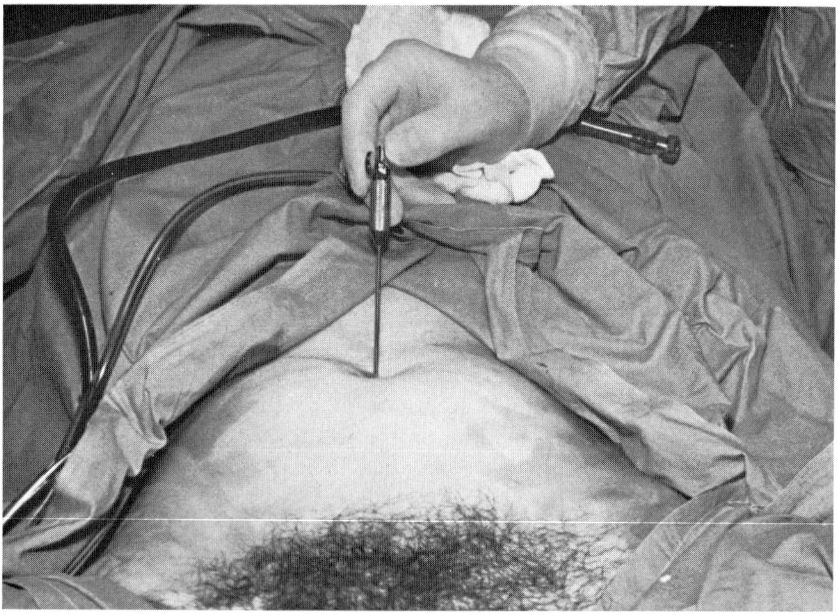

*Figure 3–2.* Verres needle insertion through periumbilical area of abdominal wall. (See Chapter 5.)

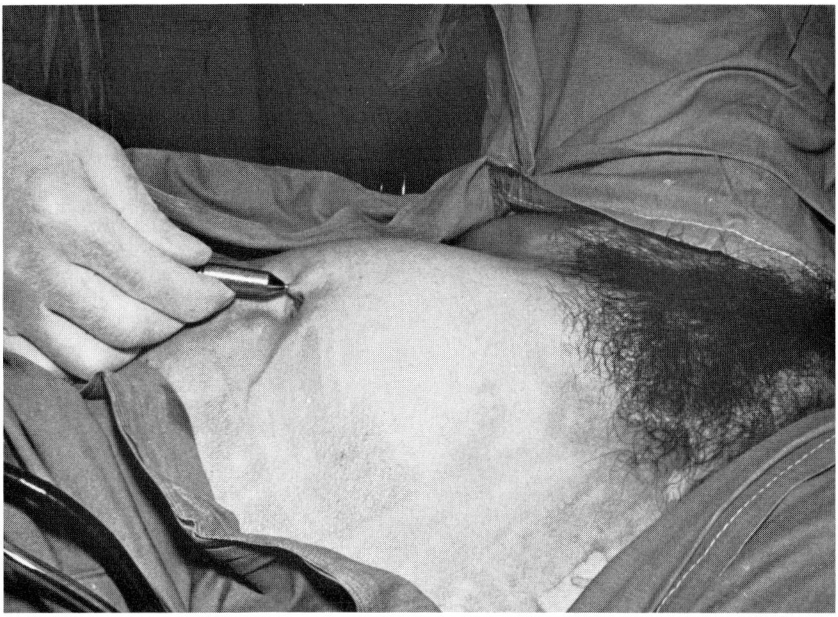

*Figure 3–3.* Abdomen distended with $CO_2$ gas.

mining the amount of gas introduced. A detailed discussion of the technique of pneumoperitoneum is presented in Chapter 5.

An incision, approximately 1 cm. in length, is placed just below or preferably to the left side of the umbilical area (Fig. 3–4). Other sites for incision are similar to those described for needle puncture (Chapter 5). For the best cosmetic results we make two tiny skin perforations with the tip of a trochar blade #12. This area is elevated with skin hooks. The umbilical area must be scrupulously clean. With the elevation of the skin near the umbilicus, a small incision is made with the trochar blade through the skin and fascia (Fig. 3–5). This tiny incision usually bleeds very little.

The trochar and valve sleeve are then inserted, first subcutaneously (Fig. 3–6) so that a good gaseous seal may be obtained, and then thrust boldly through the remaining layers of the abdominal wall into the peritoneal cavity (Fig. 3–7). The direction taken by the trochar and sleeve should be approximately 45° toward the concavity of the pelvis. The layer of gas protects the sharp trochar from damaging the intra-abdominal organs. The trochar is then removed and the valve in the sleeve closes automatically, preventing the escape of gas. To determine that the valved sleeve is in proper position, it is only necessary to depress the valve to allow a sudden escape of gas from the peritoneal cavity. The plastic tube from the source of carbon dioxide is attached to the stopcock on the valved cannula; constant

*Text continues on page 21*

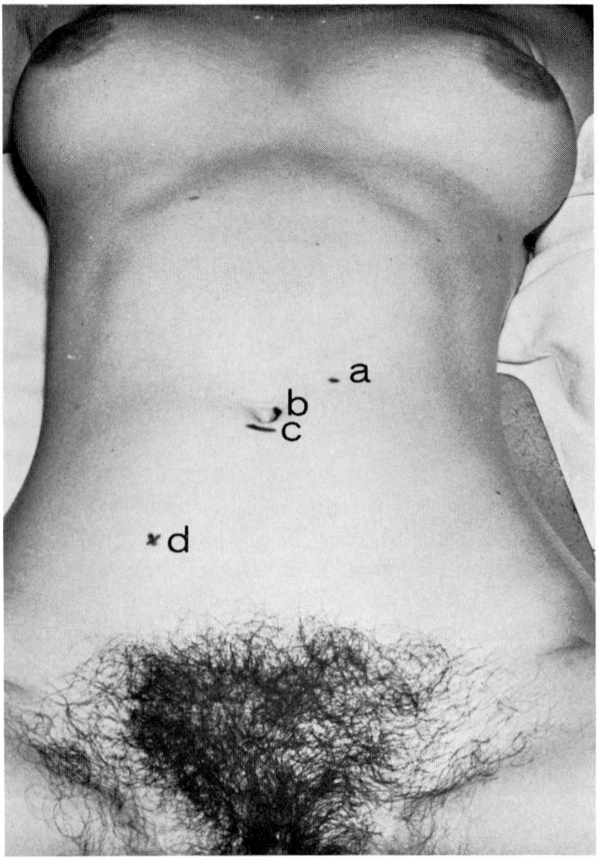


*Figure 3–4.* Abdomen marked for orientation of puncture and incision sites: (*a*) safe site for pneumoperitoneum needle. Optional incision site if sites *b* and *c* are adjacent to laparotomy scars; (*b*) typical site for needle puncture and incision; (*c*) infraumbilical site; (*d*) site for second trochar and cannula, used only after laparoscopy is in progress with adequate pneumoperitoneum.

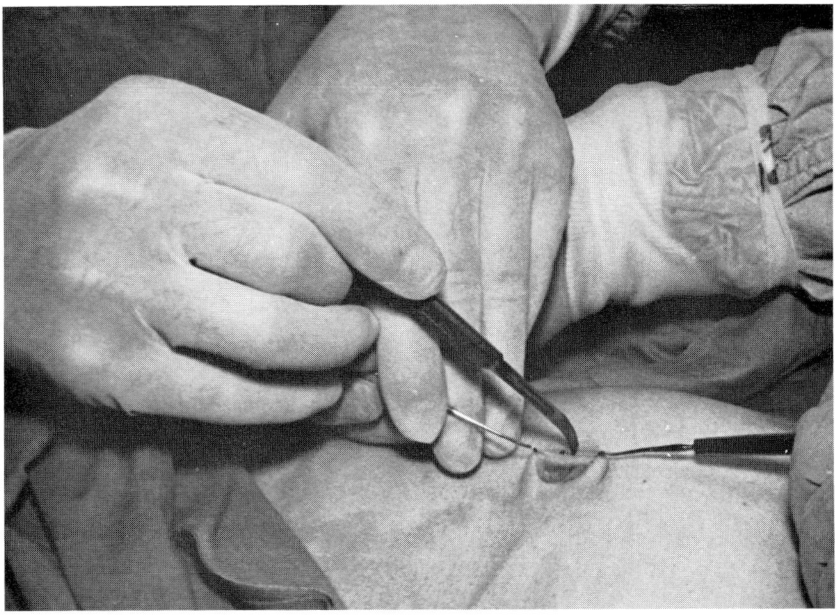

*Figure 3–5.* Lateral umbilical incision made with help of skin hooks.

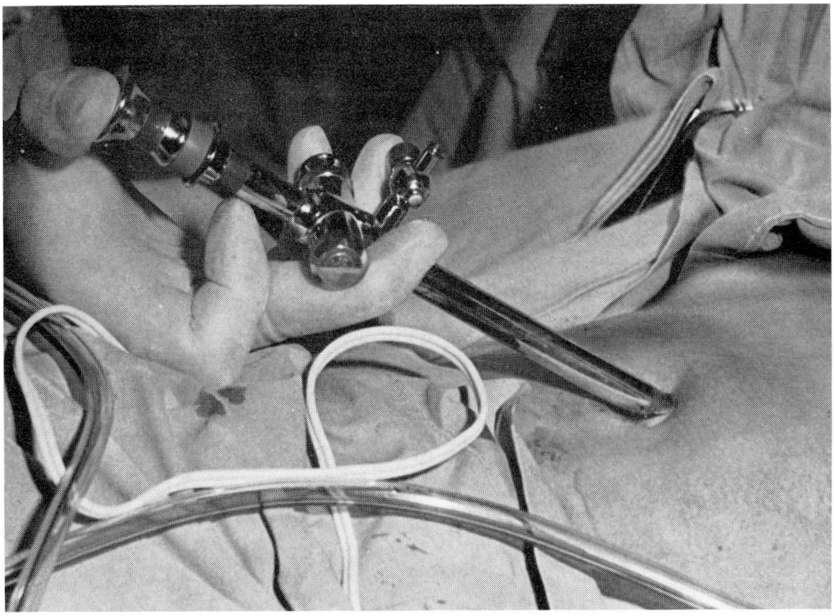

*Figure 3–6.* The trochar and cannula inserted through miniature abdominal wall incision. Direction of insertion is 45° from the horizontal toward the pelvis.

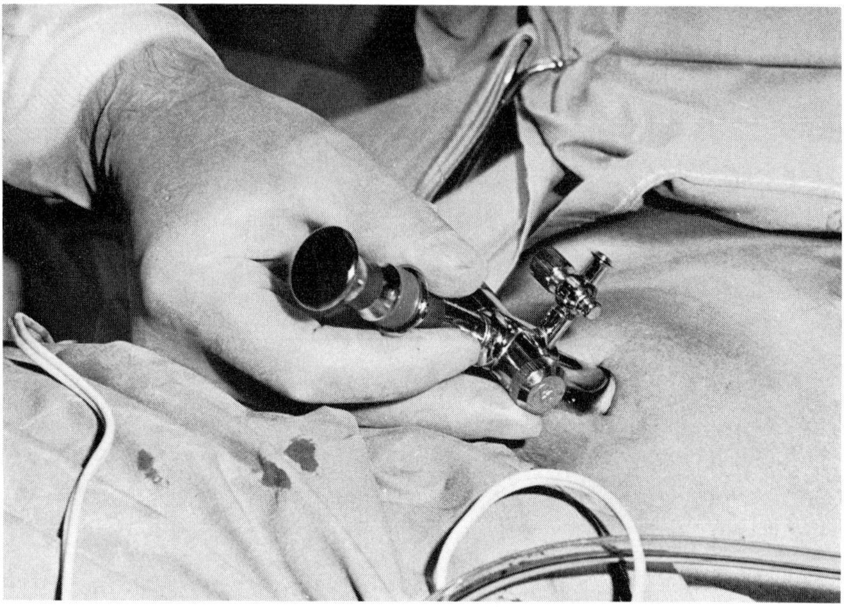

*Figure 3–7.* Insertion of trochar and cannula completed.

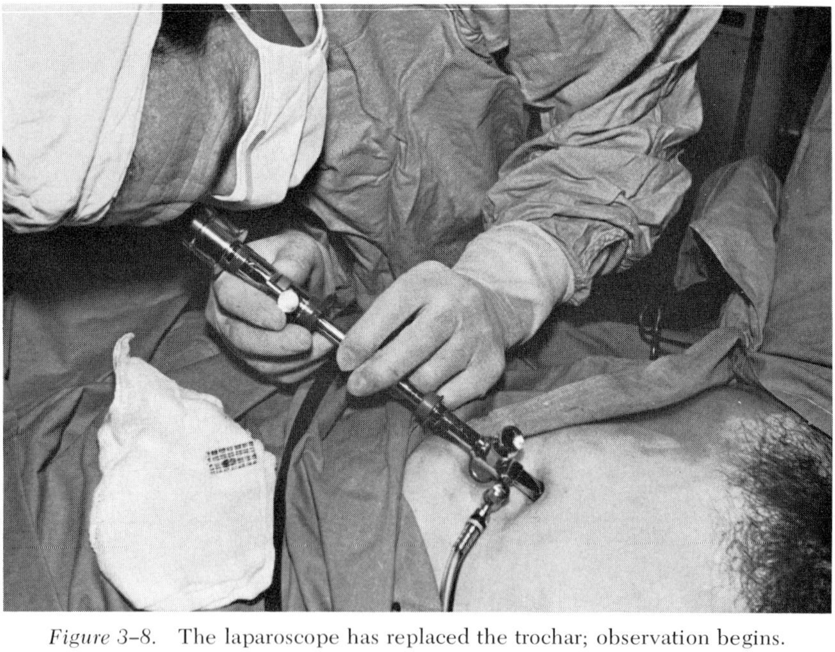

*Figure 3–8.* The laparoscope has replaced the trochar; observation begins.

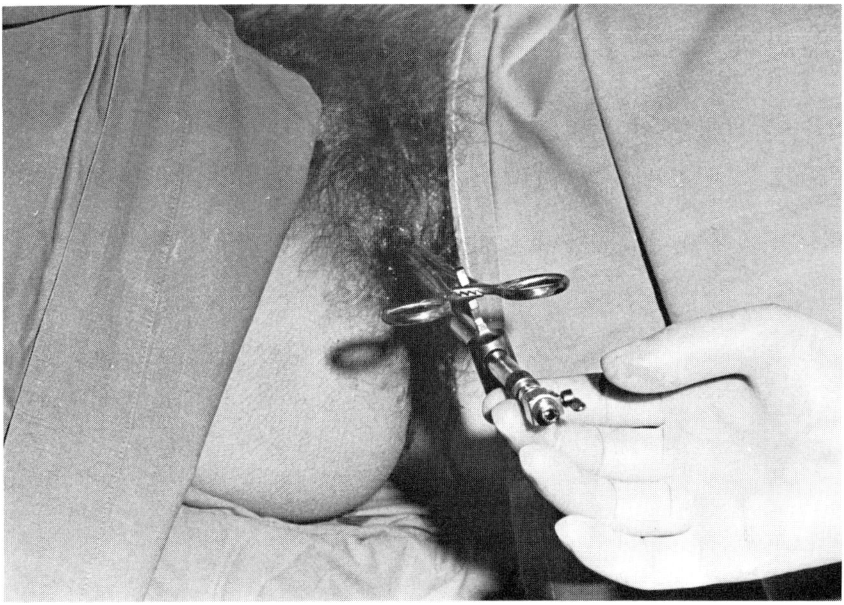

*Figure 3–9.* Uterine patency cannula hooked into position for manipulation.

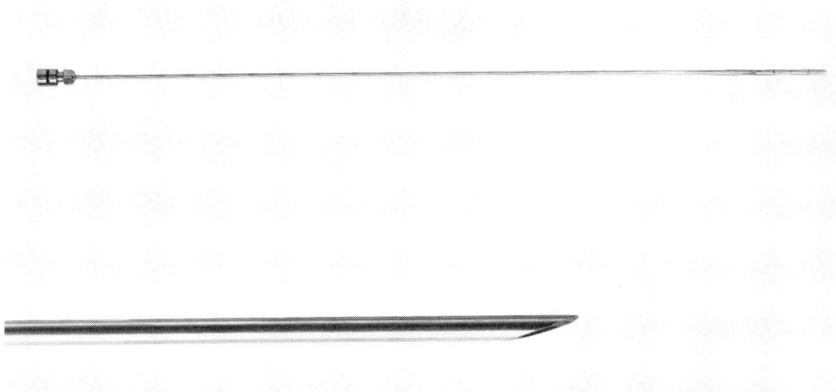

*Figure 3-10.* Behrman-Eder long needle and graduated probe (marked in centimeters) useful for manipulation and measurement.

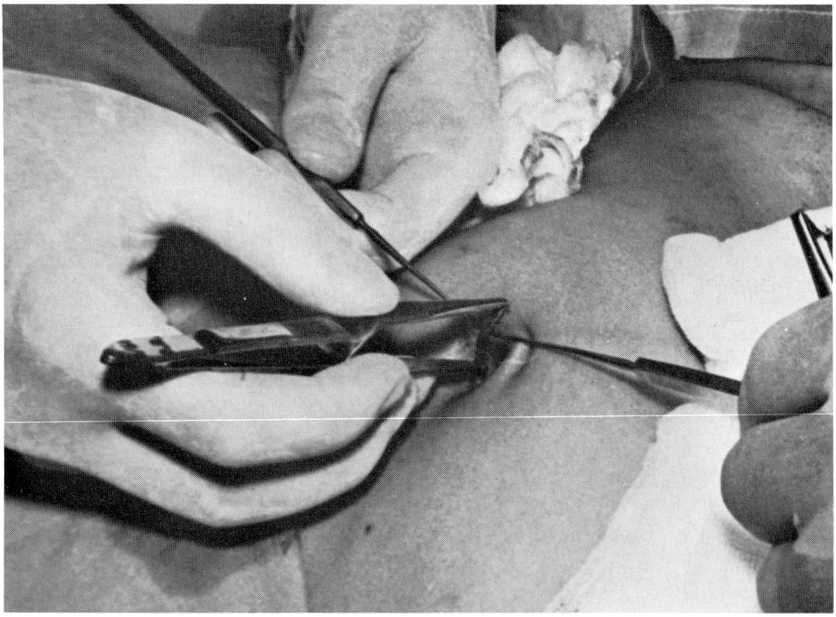

*Figure 3–11.* Skin clip closure of incision.

replacement of carbon dioxide is necessary as it is absorbed or escapes slowly from the peritoneal cavity. The laparoscope may then be introduced, the fiber optic cord attached, and inspection begun in a darkened room (Fig. 3–8).

Placing the patient in Trendelenburg position permits the pneumoperitoneum to displace the bowel from the pelvic organs so that these are readily observed. Manipulation of the intra-uterine cannula (Fig. 3–9) will elevate the pelvic organs so that both the posterior and the anterior surfaces of the uterus and its appendages may be clearly visualized. A probe (Fig. 3–10) may be inserted separately through the abdominal wall to manipulate and to measure the pelvic viscera.

At the conclusion of the operation, the laparoscope is removed. The cannula valve is opened to allow carbon dioxide to escape. The cannula is then removed. The incision is closed with a skin clip (Fig. 3–11).

### *Documentation of Findings*

Figure 3–12 shows the form we use to indicate what is seen at laparoscopy. The outline drawing is completed with colored pencils to illustrate our findings.

*The Fertility Institute*

PERITONEOSCOPY

Name____________________Pt. No.__________Date________
Surgeon________________Assistant____________Adm. No.________
Pre-op Diag. LMP____________Cycle Day____

L. 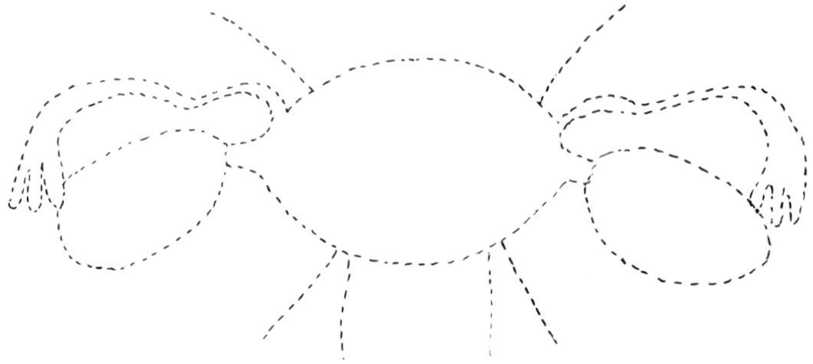 R.

PERITONEUM:
UTERUS: Size Shape Color
Abnormalities
Pathology
Uterosacral Lig.

R. OVARY: Size Shape Color Blood Vessels
Surface: Smooth Tunic Follicles
Wrinkled
Luteal Tissue
Abnormalities
Utero-Ovarian Ligament

L. OVARY: Size Shape Color Blood Vessels
Surface: Smooth Tunic Follicles
Wrinkled
Luteal Tissue
Abnormalities
Utero-Ovarian Ligament

R. TUBE: Length Color Surface
Fimbria Patency Movement Peristalsis

L. TUBE: Length Color Surface
Fimbria Patency Movement Peristalsis

PHOTOGRAPHS: Voltage Exposure Film #
Tech. Difficulty

MORBIDITY:

THERAPY:
Response:

PATHOLOGY:

*Figure 3–12.* Peritoneoscopy (laparoscopy) form.

*Chapter Four*

# ANESTHESIA FOR PELVIC LAPAROSCOPY

JULIUS H. BOLGLA, M.D.*

Anesthesia for gynecologic laparoscopy is far different from that needed for upper abdominal laparoscopy, in which we are dealing with a very ill patient, perhaps one with a liver disease or an obscure tumor. The patient is frequently advanced in years and may have other medical problems such as heart disease. These patients are usually extremely sensitive to narcotics, requiring much smaller doses than the younger patient, and local anesthesia must be used. Further, in upper abdominal laparoscopy, a lesser amount of gas is needed to create a pneumoperitoneum. In fact, when too much gas is injected, some of the visceral organs may be displaced. Also, liver disease may be associated with ascites, wherein it is very simple to remove the ascitic fluid and replace it with gas without discomfort to the patient.

The gastroenterologist usually acts as both the anesthesiologist and the endoscopist. An awake, alert patient must cooperate during upper abdominal laparoscopy because the patient's position must be constantly changed in order for the different areas in the abdomen to be seen. Local anesthesia and minimal doses of narcotics and tranquilizing drugs are usually adequate even for liver biopsy.

Gynecologic laparoscopy poses certain additional problems. First, a nonexplosive type of anesthesia must be used because (1)

*Department of Anesthesia, Michael Reese Hospital and Medical Center, Chicago, Illinois.

the power supply for both incandescent and the fiber optic scopes is electrically hazardous, (2) cautery may be used, and (3) photographic equipment is sometimes activated by means of an electronic flash.

Secondly, it is essential that a pneumoperitoneum of approximately three liters be present under pressure. The introduction of this much gas into the peritoneal cavity under pressure may cause pain, respiratory distress, and possibly cardiac embarrassment. This depends upon whether or not the patient has a relaxed abdomen, is obese, or has had children. Obviously, patients who have had children have an abdominal wall that has been previously distended, and hence they can accommodate a pneumoperitoneum with three liters of gas without a great deal of discomfort; the patient who is obese and short may have much greater difficulty. Further, Trendelenburg position is necessary so that the pelvic organs may be exposed by means of the gas. Extreme Trendelenburg position enhances respiratory and cardiac embarrassment.

The gas of choice for the pneumoperitoneum is carbon dioxide because it is readily available, rapidly absorbed, and nonexplosive. In a recent publication by Alexander et al. (1969), the effects of carbon dioxide on blood pH and $P_{CO_2}$ have been reported. The authors stated that the plasma $CO_2$ is elevated and the pH is depressed. They also reported that there is a narrowing of the pulse pressure. Siegler and Berenyi (1969) also measured the acid-base relationships in 11 patients under general anesthesia with $CO_2$ pneumoperitoneum. The control values for $P_{CO_2}$ and pH were 27.72 mm. of mercury and 7.466, respectively. At the end of laparoscopy the values for $P_{CO_2}$ and pH were 37 mm. of mercury and 7.37, respectively. It is our opinion that these changes are insignificant and would not pose any real problem during anesthesia.

Although emboli have been reported following pneumoperitoneum with carbon dioxide gas, they are more common when air is used. Other gases that can be used are nitrous oxide, which does support combustion, and oxygen, which in a sense is explosive-prone, or at least more readily supports combustion. We have had no experience with nitrogen or helium, but certainly the possibility of using such gases should be explored. The objection to nitrogen would be its slow absorption, so that the patient would complain of shoulder pain postoperatively; it is impossible to evacuate all the gas from the peritoneal cavity.

For many years the gynecologic endoscopic technique of choice at this institution has been culdoscopy. This procedure was always done under local anesthesia and hence there was little need for the anesthesia service. Laparoscopy, however, does require an experienced anesthesiologist.

Early in our experience we used general anesthesia for

laparoscopy. The technique involved premedication with meperidine and atropine sulphate. Meperidine dosage varied from 50 to 100 mg., depending on the size and age of the patient; atropine sulphate dosage was 0.4 mg. This premedication was given intramuscularly one hour preoperatively. As in any surgical procedure, an intravenous infusion of 5 per cent aqueous glucose with 0.2 per cent saline was begun. Induction of anesthesia was accomplished with sodium thiopental.* Anesthesia was then maintained with nitrous oxide and halothane† or methoxyflurane.‡ Intubation was necessary because the patient was placed in extreme Trendelenburg position and the abdomen was distended with carbon dioxide. Intubation was accomplished with succinyl choline chloride,§ 2 cc. (40 mg.) administered intravenously.

Although this anesthetic technique accomplished the objective, we felt that it was more potent than was necessary for our needs and that it subjected the patients to some unnecessary risks. The risks are postoperative pharyngeal discomfort from intubation, the possibility of liver toxicity from halothane or methoxyflurane, and the need for an additional muscle relaxant during the anesthetic procedure.

Having gained further experience in laparoscopy, we tried simplifications of the anesthetic technique. This led us to the introduction of a combination of neuroleptanalgesia¶ plus a local anesthesia.

It is essential that there be a preoperative visit with the patient. At this time the surgery and the anesthetic technique are explained, and the patient is assured that there will be very little awareness with the use of this anesthetic technique and no pain during the laparoscopy. Preoperative medication consists of 0.4 mg. atropine sulphate and 75 to 100 mg. meperidine. Currently we are exploring other preoperative medications, since there is some objection to the use of two different narcotics, viz., meperidine and fentanyl.** The latter is part of the Innovar mixture. Perhaps droperidol,†† the major tranquilizer in Innovar, plus atropine sulphate might be more ideal.

When the patient is in the operating room an intravenous infusion of 5 per cent glucose in 0.2 per cent saline is begun. The patient is placed in the lithotomy position. One per cent mepivacaine hydrochloride‡‡ is now infiltrated into the periumbilical area by the surgeon. Innovar, 5 cc. diluted to 10 cc. with physiological saline, is

*Pentothal sodium, Abbott Laboratories, North Chicago, Ill.
†Fluothane, Ayerst Laboratories, New York, N.Y.
‡Penthrane, Abbott Laboratories, North Chicago, Ill.
§Anectine, Travenol Laboratories, Morton Grove, Ill.
¶Innovar, McNeil Laboratories, Fort Washington, Pa.
**Sublimaze, McNeil Laboratories, Fort Washington, Pa.
††Inapsine, McNeil Laboratories, Fort Washington, Pa. (Not released for clinical use.)
‡‡Carbocaine, Winthrop Laboratories, New York, N.Y.

instilled slowly into the intravenous tubing until the desired state of neuroleptanalgesia is achieved. Initially, from 2 to 3 cc. of the diluted solution of Innovar is injected and the patient observed. If the state of neuroleptanalgesia is not sufficient, more of the Innovar is administered. The state of neuroleptanalgesia with optimal tranquilization usually takes eight to ten minutes to achieve. Patients usually respond satisfactorily before all 10 cc. of the diluted material is administered. Additional Innovar may be diluted and given. If the patient is still uncomfortable and not responding to Innovar, nitrous oxide and oxygen analgesia may be used supplementally.

After laparoscopy is begun, contact is maintained with the patient, who is periodically directed to breathe deeply. Patients are usually able to ventilate quite adequately without intubation even though they are in extreme Trendelenburg position and their abdomens are distended with carbon dioxide. If necessary, ventilation can be assisted with bag and mask with oxygen. The blood pressure and pulse remain stable; the patient remains dry and has good color. If laparotomy is found necessary, anesthesia is induced with nitrous oxide and oxygen, intubation is performed using 2 cc. (40 mg.) succinylcholine chloride, and anesthesia is maintained with nitrous oxide and oxygen. A mixture of Innovar, 5 cc. diluted to 20 cc., plus 1.5 cc. of succinylcholine is given intravenously in divided doses as needed.

This more complete anesthesia is entirely compatible with the neuroleptanalgesia used for laparoscopy. For the laparotomy, spinal anesthesia may be used if desired. The pneumoperitoneum at this time has been evacuated and the steep Trendelenburg position corrected.

One of the advantages of using neuroleptanalgesia for laparoscopy is that the postoperative recovery is more rapid. If laparoscopy is carried out in the morning and no further surgery is necessary, patients are ready to go home the following morning. It is inadvisable to discharge the patient the same day because the droperidol tranquilizing effect continues for 10 to 12 hours after anesthesia. It is necessary to keep the patient under observation to insure adequate ventilation. The patients are periodically encouraged to take deep breaths. We observe the usual precautions suggested for the use of neuroleptanalgesia. It is not used in patients with a history of bronchial asthma. Facilities for controlled respiration are always available, although we have not found respiratory depression to be a problem.

In summary, neuroleptanalgesia has been an entirely satisfactory technique for patients undergoing laparoscopy. It is simple to perform, depresses the patients least, and consequently permits the quickest recovery. It is compatible with deeper anesthesia if laparotomy is found to be necessary.

*Chapter Five*

# PNEUMOPERITONEUM: TECHNIQUE AND COMPLICATIONS

## TECHNIQUE

### *Site of Puncture*

The periumbilical area is the optimal site of puncture. Typically, the left side of the umbilicus is selected, inasmuch as the ligamentum teres on the right side of the umbilicus may interfere with proper insertion of the needle. Other possible sites are: (1) below the umbilicus, (2) left upper quadrant, approximately 4 cm. below the inferior costal margin, and (3) above and to the left of the umbilicus. Do not select an area adjacent to a laparotomy scar for fear of injuring the adherent bowel. Both lower quadrants should be avoided since it is possible to perforate inferior epigastric vessels; also, the needle could penetrate through the posterior parietal peritoneum into pelvic vessels or vascular fascial spaces.

### *Insertion of the Needle*

The safe introduction of gas into the peritoneal cavity requires a proper needle and a source of gas. A standard #18 gauge spinal needle may be used, but it is safer to use a needle with two stylets, one sharp and one dull. The sharp stylet is useful for perforation of the skin and superficial fascia, while the dull stylet is preferable to pierce the deep fascia, the posterior rectus sheath, and the perito-

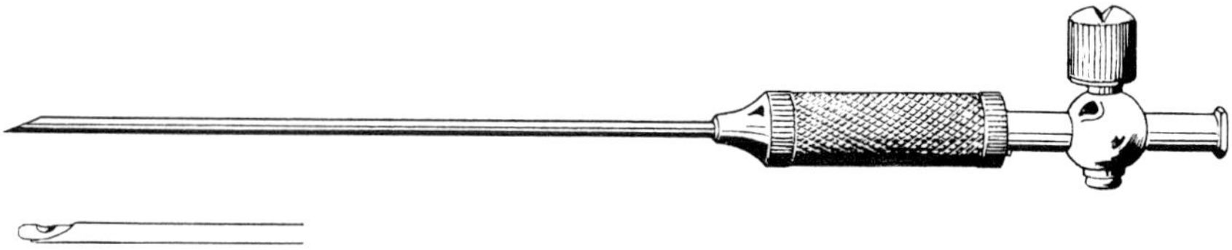

*Figure 5–1.* Verres needle, size 15 gauge and 10 cm. long.

neum. The Verres needle (Fig. 5–1) is an automatic needle with spring action that combines an outer sharp point and an inner dull stylet. The surgeon should be able to feel the needle traversing each layer of the abdominal wall. It is frequently necessary to lift the lower abdominal wall with one hand as the other hand advances the needle through the layers of the abdomen.

After the needle has been inserted into the peritoneal cavity, the following safety tests are suggested:

1. Move the needle back and forth to make sure that it is in a free space.
2. Attach a syringe, partially filled with saline, for aspiration. If the needle had entered a loop of bowel or the dilated stomach, intestinal or gastric contents with or without gas would be obtained. If a blood vessel had been entered, blood would be withdrawn. If nothing can be aspirated, the saline is injected; it should flow freely into the peritoneal cavity. Then and only then may the surgeon proceed with the injection of the gas.

### *Creating the Pneumoperitoneum*

Various gases have been used to induce a pneumoperitoneum. The original technique utilized air pumped by hand. Reports of air emboli in the early literature now indict as too hazardous the use of air for pneumoperitoneum. Oxygen, nitrogen, nitrous oxide, and carbon dioxide have all been used. Carbon dioxide is the gas of choice because it (1) does not support combustion, (2) is rapidly absorbed, and (3) is rapidly excreted. Small volumes of carbon dioxide can even be tolerated intravenously because of its rapid absorption.

A simple apparatus in use at Michael Reese Hospital (Fig. 5–2) combines a carbon dioxide tank fitted with a shutoff valve, gauge, and flowmeter. The flowmeter is calibrated in liters per minute. A manometer, similar to the type used to record blood pressure, indicates the gas pressure in the system going to the patient. This apparatus has proved satisfactory, but there are more precise insufflation machines available, namely, the instrument of Professor Semm.

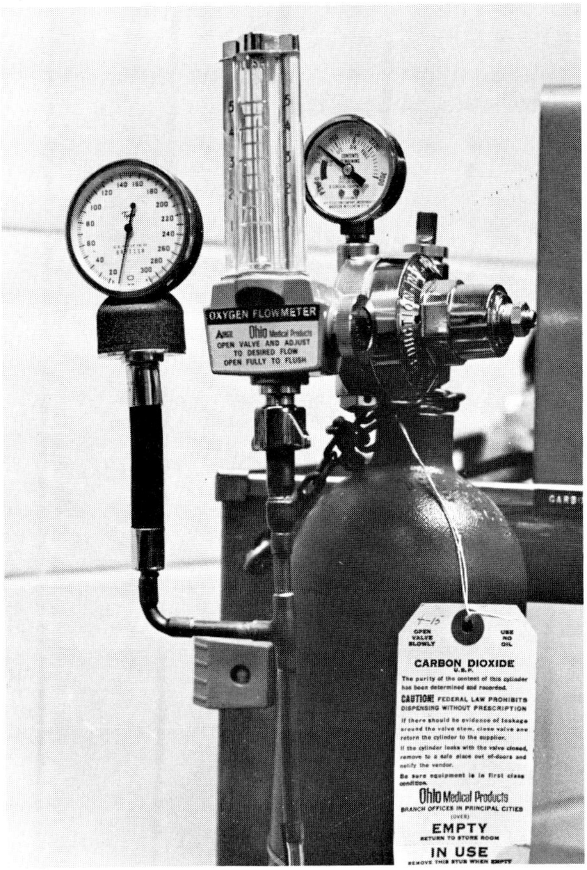


*Figure 5–2.* Carbon dioxide tank with shutoff valve and gauge, flowmeter, copper T tube, and manometer (from right to left).

**The Semm Insufflator** (Fig. 5–3). This is an instrument that is attached to a tank of carbon dioxide gas. The insufflator has a receptacle which holds five liters of carbon dioxide. Insufflation may be performed with the valve set for manual or automatic operation. Original inflation is performed manually and pressure must not exceed 40 mm. of mercury. A ball valve indicates when gas is flowing freely. An obstruction to the flow of gas is registered when pressure rises to the red area between 40 and 60 mm. of mercury, thus indicating a need for adjustment of the pneumoperitoneum needle.

After the needle is introduced, plastic tubing from the source of carbon dioxide gas is attached to the valve of the needle, and a trial insufflation is made under low pressure. One must be aware of the inherent resistance of gas flowing through the needle so that a gas pressure just above this primary resistance can be established. That is, if a pressure of 20 mm. of mercury is necessary for gas to traverse the Verres needle, the gas flow would necessarily be increased to 30 or 40 mm. of mercury. During the insufflation the pressure must be carefully monitored. If necessary, the needle should be rotated or otherwise advanced or withdrawn slightly to allow free flow of gas.

Whether an automatic or homemade apparatus is used, it is very important to watch the pressure gauge carefully. Gas under high pressure should never be injected into the peritoneal cavity. It must be remembered that most of the complications in laparoscopy have occurred during the induction of pneumoperitoneum.

As the gas begins to flow into the peritoneal cavity, it is helpful to percuss the abdomen to determine whether a pneumoperitoneum is being produced. It is important to ascertain that gas is present in the upper as well as in the lower abdomen. Liver dullness typically disappears. After sufficient distention has been obtained, the needle is withdrawn.

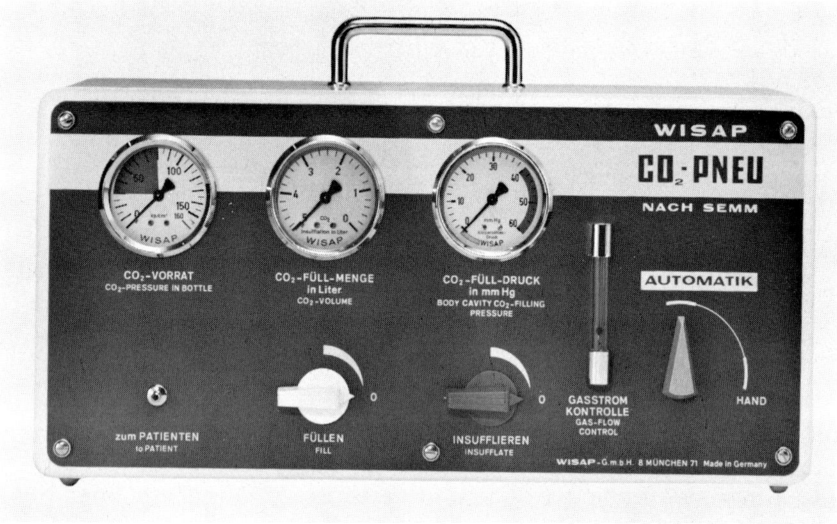


*Figure* 5–3. The Semm insufflator. The *left upper* gauge indicates $CO_2$ pressure in the $CO_2$ tank. The valve marked "FILL," when opened to + (obscured by valve handle in photograph), allows gas to a capacity of five liters to enter a storage tank. When this tank is filled, the needle of the middle gauge points to 0. The middle gauge is the volume meter. The *right upper* gauge indicates the amount of pressure created during insufflation when the valve marked "INSUFFLATE" is turned to +. The pressure gauge should not reach the dark (red) area between 40 and 60 mm. of mercury. The *right lower* valve is turned to "HAND" during insufflation. After approximately three liters of gas has been delivered to create the initial pneumoperitoneum, this valve is turned to "AUTOMATIK" and the tank is refilled (middle gauge to 0). The glass tube marked "GAS-FLOW CONTROL" contains a black ball that rises when there is a free flow of $CO_2$ into the peritoneal cavity.

Women who have had one or more babies usually have a flaccid, easily distensible abdominal wall and may tolerate large quantities of gas. In contradistinction, the nulliparous patient, especially one who is shortwaisted or obese, tolerates much smaller quantities of gas. After a pneumoperitoneum has been established, it is possible to test whether the gas is in the right place by aspirating through the abdominal wall with a long needle and syringe. In the early experience with the technique of laparoscopy, patients were selected only from those with an abdomen distended with ascites. In this situation it was very simple to remove the ascitic fluid and substitute gas. However, most gynecologic patients have no ascites, and the establishment of a pneumoperitoneum is more difficult and critical. When approximately three liters of gas have been inserted into the peritoneal cavity, the trochar and trochar sleeve may be safely inserted into the peritoneal cavity.

## COMPLICATIONS

If the pneumoperitoneal needle is not sufficiently long or if, during the introduction of gas, it slips back into the layers of the abdominal wall, gas may accumulate either in the subcutaneous tissue or between the layers of fascia and peritoneum. This is not a serious complication since carbon dioxide is absorbed very quickly and may be very simply evacuated. On rare occasions, after establishment of what is thought to be a pneumoperitoneum, it soon becomes apparent that one has entered a tissue space rather than the free peritoneal cavity. When this occurs, the gas is evacuated and an attempt at pneumoperitoneum is again made. Subcutaneous gas may possibly extend as far as the area of the neck and inguinal regions.

It is possible for the needle to injure some small blood vessels and to produce a hematoma of the abdominal wall. We once encountered a large hematoma of the abdominal wall that was associated with intraperitoneal blood. It necessitated immediate laparotomy to find the source of the bleeding and ligation of the vessel in the abdominal wall.

If one of the loops of the bowel is adherent to the parietal peritoneum, the gas may be injected into the lumen of bowel. This is not a very serious complication since the gas may be easily expelled. It is also possible for the needle to penetrate the omentum and produce emphysema. Occasionally one sees omenta distended with vesicles of gas, but this is usually a benign complication and the gas is absorbed very rapidly. Blood vessels in the omentum conceivably might be injured and produce a hematoma. In our series this has never happened. It is possible for a needle to penetrate the liver or spleen, but this is highly unlikely in gynecologic laparoscopy.

When overdistention of the abdomen and elevation of the diaphragm occurs, compression of the heart and great vessels could result in transient shock; this is relieved by releasing gas from the peritoneal cavity. Under light anesthesia, such as a local plus neuroleptanalgesia, the patient herself is aware of overdistention of the abdomen and she is alert enough to complain of abdominal tightness or pain. As a result of increased abdominal pressure, the abdominal contour may disclose hernial sacs in the inguinal region. This also is an error in technique. Much care is advised in employing laparoscopy in a patient with known inguinal or umbilical hernias. In a patient with a diaphragmatic or hiatus hernia this procedure must be performed with a great deal of caution, if at all.

*Chapter Six*

# THE LAPAROSCOPE AND OTHER EQUIPMENT

## THE LAPAROSCOPE AND POWER SUPPLY

The laparoscope (Figs. 6–1, 6–2, 6–3, and 6–4) is a rigid instrument varying in diameter from 4 mm. to 10 mm.; it incorporates an optical system plus a means of illumination. The optical system employs glass optics and focusing of the laparoscope is not necessary. The objective of the scope is directed forward 180° or foroblique 135°. This differs from the culdoscope which is directed at a 90° angle. The scope must be long enough to reach from the midabdomen down into the pelvis or up to the upper abdominal regions as needed. Optimally, its length should be 300 mm. In older scopes an incandescent lighting system is present, and hence a power source or battery is required to illuminate the 4 to 6 volt lamp placed at the end of the scope. Incandescent scopes are always foroblique in design.

Modern illumination systems are provided with fiber optics incorporated in the laparoscope. The modus operandi of fiber optics (cold light) is illustrated in Figure 6–5. Each manufacturer of laparoscopes provides fiber optic power sources, all of which are based upon the same principle of a projector-type bulb housed in an air-cooled box. A lens system focuses the light at the proximal tip of the fiber optic bundle, which varies in length from 4 to 6 feet. The transmitted light, as it enters and leaves the laparoscope, is cold. Sufficient illumination for viewing requires no more than a standard 150 watt projection bulb. Photography requires more powerful light,

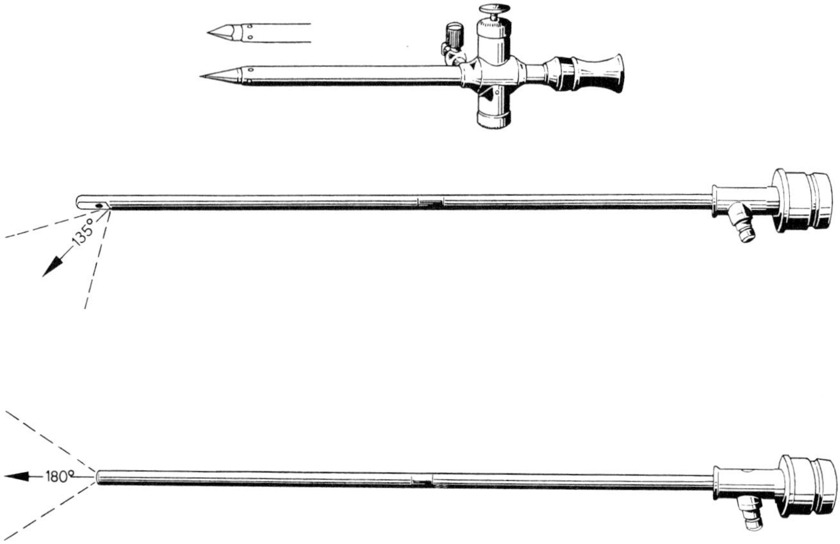


*Figure 6–1.* Valved cannula and trochar with Frangenheim laparoscopes. Manufactured by Richard Wolf, Knittlingen, West Germany; distributed by AGA Corporation, Secaucus, N.J. and Eder Instrument Company, Chicago, Ill. From top down: pyramidal tip and conical tip trochars, 135° foroblique, and 180° direct forward laparoscopes.

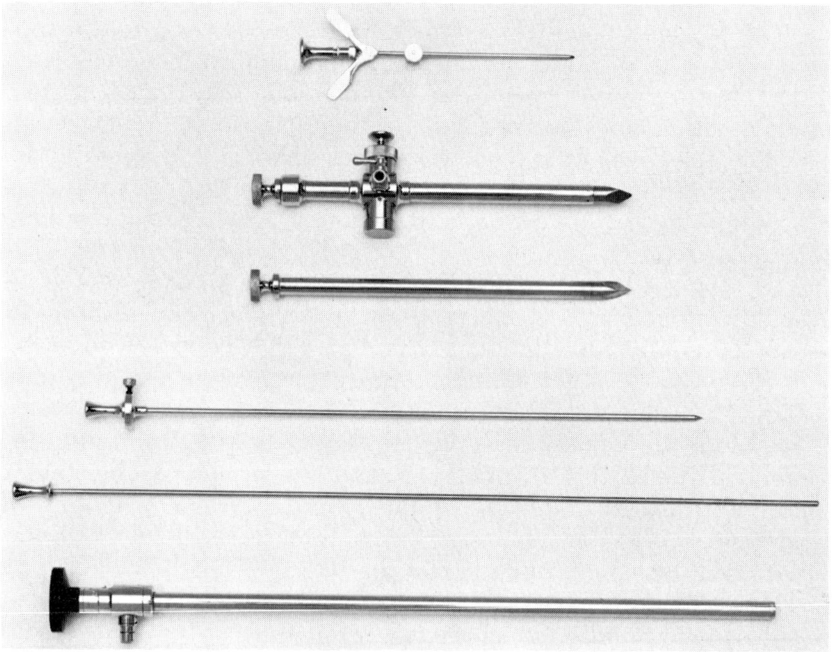

*Figure 6–2.* A.C.M.I. laparoscope, manufactured by American Cystoscope Makers, Inc., Pelham, N.Y. From top down: pneumoperitoneum needle (Ruddock), main cannula and trochars (blunt and sharp trochars), secondary cannula and trochar with graduated probe, and examining direct vision telescope.

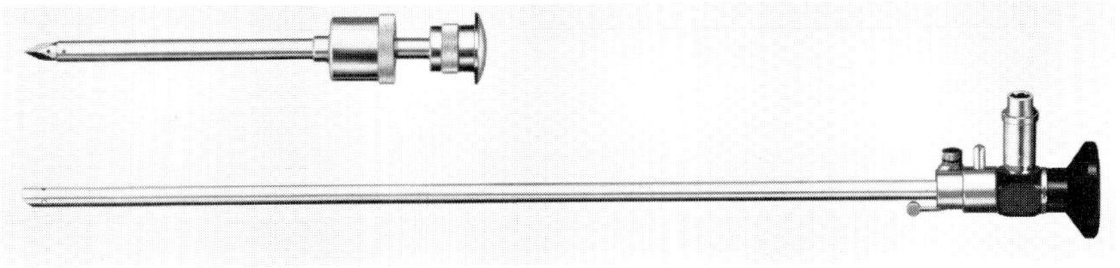

*Figure 6–3.* Hopkins laparoscope (diam. 4 mm.) with trochar and valved cannula. Manufactured by Storz Instrument Company, St. Louis, Mo.

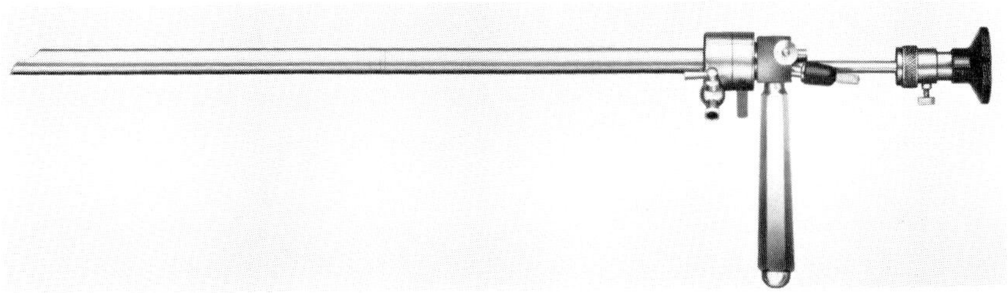

*Figure 6–4.* "Universal" peritoneoscope (Menghini-Wildhirt's). Manufactured by Storz Instrument Company, St. Louis, Mo.

e.g., the 1000 watt General Electric lamp incorporated in the Eder 1000 power supply (Fig. 6–6). Two portable fiber optic power supplies are illustrated in Figures 6–7 and 6–8.

In the new 180° laparoscope, the objective lens is at the tip of the scope and is surrounded by fiber optic light fibers. This is a very popular instrument, although the optical system is more apt to become clouded when the tip of the scope touches intraperitoneal organs. Frequently the scope has to be removed from the peritoneal cavity, the optics cleaned, and the instrument reinserted.

The foroblique instrument has a tip, projecting approximately 1 to 2 cm., that may be used as a probe. With this instrument soiling of the objective lens is less likely.

## THE TROCHAR AND VALVED CANNULA

The trochar is of the same diameter as the laparoscope. It fits into the valved cannula when the valve is depressed and it extends about 1 to 1.5 cm. beyond the end of the cannula so that it may be easily thrust into the peritoneal cavity after creation of the pneumoperitoneum. The tip of the trochar may either be conical or pyramidal. The pyramidal tip, which is preferred, has a three-edged point with surfaces ground concavely for greater ease of penetration through the abdominal wall.

The diameter of the valved cannula is usually about 1 mm. greater than the diameter of the trochar or the laparoscope. The

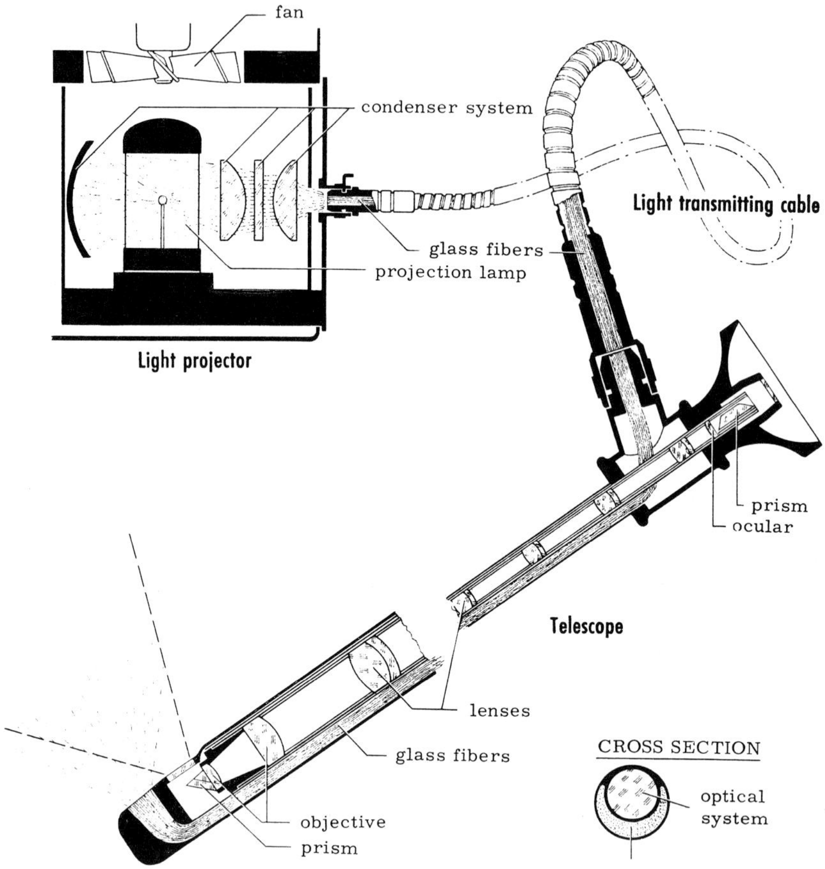


Figure 6–5. Diagram of fiber optic light supply to laparoscope. In this illumination system light from a separate light source (projector) is transmitted via a detachable, flexible light cable to the instrument and via a conductor of glass fibers inside the instrument to the distal end. This means that illumination is not accomplished by a small tungsten lamp as formerly. The heat produced by the lamp is mainly eliminated by a filter; the rest is absorbed by the fibers so that an actual cold light leaves the distal end of the instrument. Excessive heating of the condenser system and of the lamp is avoided by means of a fan.

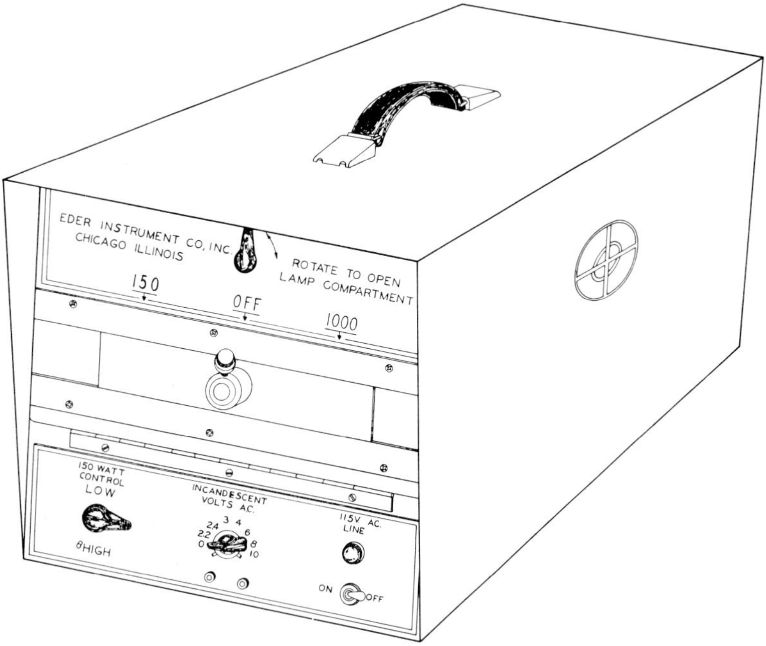


*Figure 6-6.* Power supply for routine endoscopy as well as for photography. Manufactured by Eder Instrument Company, Chicago, Ill. Two light sources are available, 150 and 1000 watts, respectively, for transmittal through the fiber optic bundle of the laparoscope. Selection is made by merely sliding the center panel to the left (150 watts) or to the right (1000 watts).

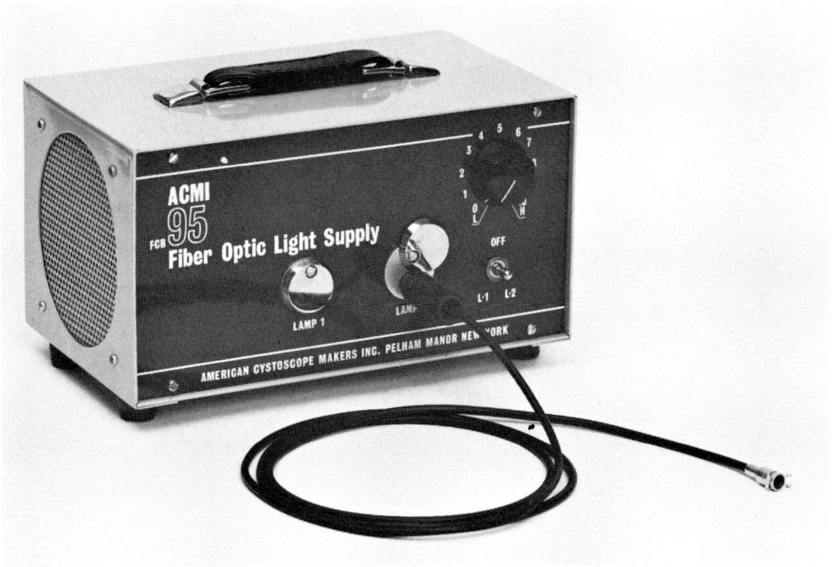


*Figure 6-7.* Portable dual lamp unit, manufactured by American Cystoscope Makers, Inc., Pelham, N.Y.

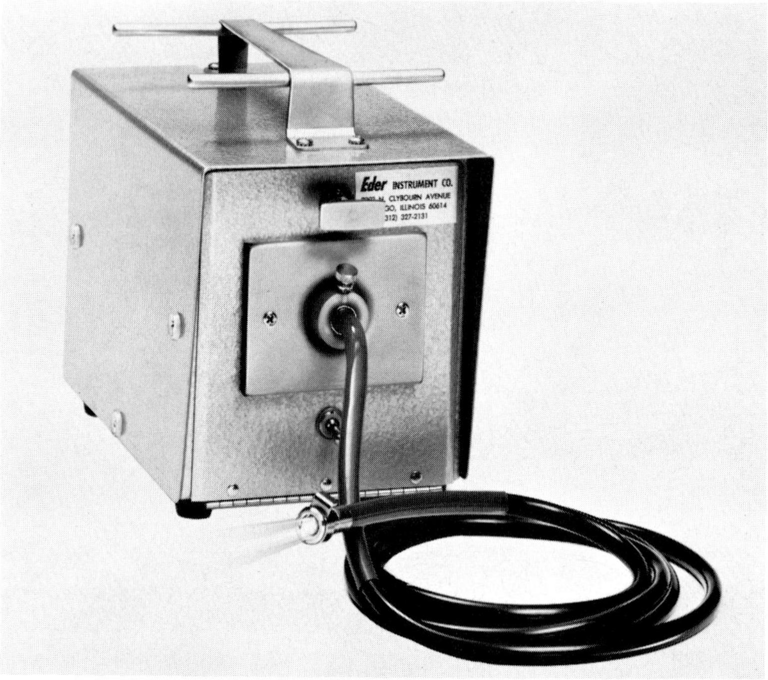


*Figure 6–8.* Portable fiber optic power supply with new General Electric EKN 17.5 v., 120 watt lamp. This new lamp is cooler and lasts 130 hours. Manufactured by Eder Instrument Company, Chicago, Ill.

cannula is a simple hollow tube incorporating a valve, much like a trumpet valve, that is necessary to prevent the escape of intraperitoneal gas when the laparoscope is exchanged for the trochar. Distal to the valve is a stopcock; tubing from the source of carbon dioxide may be attached here. At the end of the cannula are perforations which allow the release of gas through the cannula to replace gas lost or absorbed during the laparoscopic procedure.

### *Fogging of Optics*

To prevent the optics from fogging in the warm, moist peritoneal cavity, it is necessary to warm the instruments before insertion. In addition to warming, we use an antifogging detergent, hexachlorophene.* Warming the scopes is mandatory with the newer 180° fiber optic scope because the glass optics are surrounded and insulated by fiber optic bundles transmitting light. (The 135° inandescent scope does not fog as readily.) The instrument is dipped

*Septisol, Vestal Laboratory, Inc., St. Louis, Mo.

in 99° F. water and dried carefully; the lens is moistened with hexachlorophene, wiped dry, and immediately inserted through the valved cannula into the peritoneal cavity. Instead of warm water, a source of dry heat may be utilized. Friction with a dry surgical sponge is also effective in warming the cold tip of the laparoscope. Should the lens still fog, it is necessary to remove the scope for rewarming and recleaning of the lens. The lens must be crystal clear, and visualization should be so exact that every blood vessel may be seen.

### *Cleaning and Sterilization of Instruments*

The modern laparoscopist is blessed with the availability of fine optical instruments, which must be kept clean and in good working order. The physician must be familiar with the mechanics of the valved cannula and be able to take it apart for cleaning and lubrication. The cannula must be cleaned with a nylon brush, detergent, and clear rinses. The rubber gasket, which prevents undue leakage of gas from the peritoneal cavity, must be inspected and replaced if it shows signs of deterioration. The Verres needle can be disassembled and cleaned thoroughly. The laparoscope is simply cleaned and dried with a soft cloth to avoid scratching the lens.

The instruments are usually gas sterilized; they are *never* autoclaved. However, when more than one endoscopic procedure is performed, it may be necessary to cold sterilize the instruments in activated dialdehyde* for ten minutes. The instruments are then carefully rinsed in at least two rinses of sterile water. It is important to dry the instruments very carefully since any moisture will fog the lenses. When the valved cannula is placed in the cold sterilizing solution, it is necessary to activate the valve so that the solution will enter the cannula. Likewise, when the cannula is rinsed in sterile water the valve again must be activated to release the antiseptic solution. Physicians have complained about smarting of their eyes because of formaldehyde gas, while performing laparoscopy. This is due to improperly rinsed instruments after cold sterilization

*Cidex, Arbrook, Somerville, N.J.

*Chapter Seven*

# INDICATIONS AND CONTRAINDICATIONS FOR LAPAROSCOPY

## INDICATIONS

Although laparoscopy dates back to Kelling (1901), and literally hundreds of papers have been written about it, the technique is new to American gynecologists. Indications for this endoscopic procedure are slowly evolving. The gynecologist with experience in culdoscopy will find that the indications for laparoscopy are similar. Laparoscopy is indicated in obscure pelvic complaints, for which the standard methods of pelvic examination, x-ray, or other laboratory examinations are inconclusive, and when laparotomy is contemplated.

Laparoscopy is a visual technique and interpretation depends upon familiarity with gross anatomy and pathology. In addition, it is possible to perform ancillary procedures, such as aspiration of cysts or peritoneal fluid, and biopsy. Our chief indications for this examination have been in suspected ectopic pregnancy and as part of the evaluation of the infertile female. In the future, indications for laparoscopy may be extended. Our guiding principle is whether direct inspection and possible biopsy is of sufficient diagnostic value to warrant hospitalization and anesthesia, plus this minor surgical technique.

In the differential diagnosis between appendicitis and salpingitis it may or may not be helpful. If an overt pelvic peritonitis is present, laparoscopy may even be dangerous because a matted bowel may be present and obstruct the view of the pelvic organs. Possible bowel injury might occur during attempts at visualization. Further, the appendix is only visible when it is anterior and free in the peritoneal cavity. The retrocecal appendix is not visible.

As a rule, we advise either culdoscopy or laparoscopy in all patients who have been infertile for a period of three years or longer, or who are thirty years of age or older. It can be very useful in patients for whom the standard techniques of evaluation, such as the Rubin test, hysterosalpingography, and ovulation timing, are inconclusive. It can also be useful in diagnosing amenorrhea.

Besides the usefulness of this technique for unexplained infertility, it should be employed prior to contemplated surgery, especially tubal plastic operations. Further, we advise that it be routinely employed six months later to evaluate the results of such surgery and to see whether adhesions have re-formed. This second look, which presents the possibility of lysis of small adhesions under endoscopic control, is of value not only to the patient, but also to the surgeon who is constantly striving to improve his operative technique. We have also found laparoscopy useful in evaluating the effects of drugs, especially those used in stimulating ovulation.

## CONTRAINDICATIONS

Laparoscopy is contraindicated in:

1. Patients for whom anesthesia would be contraindicated. Although it is possible to do the procedure under local anesthesia, it is frequently necessary to employ general anesthesia in gynecologic laparoscopy. Certainly patients with serious heart or pulmonary diseases would be excluded.
2. Intestinal obstruction or peritonitis.
3. Extensive herniations, especially those with hiatus hernia.
4. Extensive abdominal scarring from prior laparotomies.
5. Patients with a history of peritonitis in whom one might expect extensive bowel adhesions.

When it is impossible to establish pneumoperitoneum safely, the technique is contraindicated.

Age per se is not a contraindication; most patients in our series were in their twenties or thirties. The very young patient requires general anesthesia; the very old patient does well with local anesthesia plus narcosis, neuroleptanalgesia, or tranquilizing drugs.

*Chapter Eight*

# COMPLICATIONS OF LAPAROSCOPY

Complications of laparoscopy may be due to (1) anesthesia, (2) the induction of the pneumoperitoneum, (3) the introduction of the trochar and trochar sleeve, (4) the laparoscope, and (5) the performance of ancillary techniques.

Regarding anesthesia, one must make certain that preoperative medications are adequate, that overdosage is avoided, and that the patient is not allergic to the medication. Complications from general anesthesia are rare. However, an experienced anesthesiologist should be entrusted with this part of the procedure. (See Chapter 4.)

Minor complications inherent in producing a pneumoperitoneum have already been discussed in Chapter 5. Major complications from pneumoperitoneum have not occurred in our series.

## COMPLICATIONS DUE TO THE INTRODUCTION OF THE TROCHAR AND TROCHAR SLEEVE

If a proper pneumoperitoneum has been established, the insertion of the trochar and trochar sleeve should not produce any complications. There is the rare likelihood that this sharp instrument could perforate the bowel or injure the abdominal wall or omental blood vessels resulting in intra-abdominal or intraperitoneal hemorrhage. All gynecologists performing this technique should be prepared to do an immediate laparotomy should such a rare complication occur. If there is even a suspicion of bowel injury, laparotomy is mandatory. It is suggested in such cases that the instruments be left in place while laparotomy is being performed so that the point of perforation can be easily identified and repair accomplished. Bowel complication has not occurred in our series of over 500 laparoscopic examinations. A mild abdominal wall hematoma requires no treatment, but an extensive abdominal hematoma must be evacuated and the bleeding point secured.

## COMPLICATIONS DUE TO THE LAPAROSCOPE

There is a possibility of producing damage with the laparoscope itself. In our series, trauma to a vascular corpus luteum produced sufficient intra-abdominal hemorrhage to necessitate laparotomy and control of the ovarian bleeding point.

When taking still photographs we use the Richard Wolf scope with incandescent lighting and an electronic flash and we have had no complications. However, I would insist that less experienced surgeons use the fiber optic (cold light) laparoscope rather than one with an incandescent bulb which might overheat and produce internal burn injury.

## COMPLICATIONS DUE TO THE PERFORMANCE OF ANCILLARY TECHNIQUES

Damage to adjacent organs or hemorrhage could ensue with ancillary techniques of biopsy, tubal sterilization, or aspiration of cysts. It is also possible that techniques of lysis of adhesions with an electrocautery may be followed by late complications due to sloughing. Therefore, it is mandatory that the endoscopist garner sufficient experience using visual techniques only before employing these ancillary procedures. We personally have had no complications following lysis of adhesions nor have complications occurred in any of our 50 interval sterilizations via laparoscopy. (See Chapter 10.)

## COMPLICATIONS OF LAPAROSCOPY REPORTED IN THE LITERATURE

Kalk and Wildhirt (1962) reported two fatal complications out of 60,129 cases. One was a patient suffering from liver cirrhosis, in whom the trochar injured a sclerotic vein in the abdominal wall. The other fatality was a patient suffering from serious cardiac decompensation. The patient died during induction of the pneumoperitoneum. Reports of these and other fatalities are given in Table 8–1. Nonfatal complications included: perforation of the colon adherent to the abdominal wall (three cases, all of which healed without operative intervention), omental hematoma, hematoma of the abdominal wall, pneumocolon (four cases), right-sided pneumothorax, cutaneous emphysema extending to the neck, mediastinal emphysema, and cutaneous emphysema (an incidence of 2.2 per thousand).

Fervers (1933) employed cautery in the presence of an oxygen pneumoperitoneum. Explosion occurred intra-abdominally, but the patient was not injured.

In his series of 900 cases Ruddock (1939) reported nine complications and one death. The complications were: small bowel perforations (four cases with operative repair in three of these), colon puncture (two cases with repair), stomach puncture from the pneumoperitoneum needle (surgical repair required), and stomach perforation with trochar (repair of perforation required). The single death occurred in a patient with extensive metastatic carcinoma of the liver in which hemorrhage followed biopsy of a nodule. Ruddock reported only three unsuccessful examinations due to abdominal wall adhesions. He preferred the infra-umbilical approach; after the needle was inserted, it was moved around in a circle to determine the presence of adhesions or a fixed bowel at the point of entry.

Ruddock (1949) reported two additional fatalities in a series of 2500 patients. One followed biopsy of the spleen with brisk hemorrhage; the patient died during splenectomy. The second patient had ascites; the peritoneoscopy incision was left open for drainage, permitting a tongue of omentum to protrude. Laparotomy was followed by generalized peritonitis and death.

Shackelford (1941) described two cases of intestinal perforation with recovery.

Vilardell et al. (1968) reported 1455 cases performed from 1936 to 1968 at the School of Gastro-enterology. Complications occurred in 18 patients (1.2 per cent) and included severe subcutaneous emphysema, pneumothorax, bowel puncture, gallbladder perforation, colon perforation, and abdominal hemorrhage. They reported two deaths (0.13 per cent) (Table 8–1).

### *Air Emboli*

At one time artificial pneumoperitoneum was very important in the treatment of pulmonary tuberculosis. Today chemotherapy and lung surgery have replaced this method. However, reports of complications of pneumoperitoneum in the medical literature are still of interest.

Banyai (1946) stated that air embolism was the most serious

complication of pneumoperitoneum and that it occurs most frequently during the physician's early experience with this treatment.

Dasher et al. (1954), in a review of complications of artificial pneumoperitoneum for the treatment of tuberculosis, reported 127 cases of air emboli with 74 fatalities. In their own series, among 1800 patients who had more than 80,000 refills there were only two fatalities due to air embolism. In addition, they reported three nonfatal cases.

Hartleib (1955) reported two fatalities due to lung embolism during laparoscopy. In both cases pneumoperitoneum was produced through the right side of the abdomen at a distance of a few centimeters below the costal arch. One patient died suddenly after the introduction of only 30 ml. of air. The autopsy findings revealed that the pneumoperitoneum needle had penetrated the right lobe of an enlarged liver. The air was pumped into the liver, then traveled through its veins and the inferior vena cava to the heart and lungs.

Wenderoth (1954), in a discussion of Hartleib's report, stressed that the emboli were not caused by the pneumoperitoneum, but rather by introducing a needle directly into liver veins. He criticized Hartleib's site of insertion of the pneumoperitoneum needle in the right upper abdomen. He doubted that 30 cc. of air was sufficient to cause death and cited experiments demonstrating that from 10 to 100 cc. of air may be injected intravenously without causing serious problems. However, it is theoretically possible that small amounts of air could get to the brain through a patent foramen ovale with a fatal outcome. Wenderoth quotes Maier (1939) who extracted 80 cc. of air from the right ventricle with recovery of the patient.

### *Pneumothorax*

Riegel (1952) described two cases of pneumothorax during laparoscopy. According to Riegel, pneumothorax during laparoscopy can develop because of (a) developmental anomalies with thin dehiscences in the diaphragm, (b) a pathologic condition such as tuberculosis of the diaphragm, or (c) increased abdominal pressure plus pulmonary emphysema. He attributed his first case to tuberculosis and the second to emphysema.

Motschmann (1954) reported right-sided pneumothorax that developed during laparoscopy; he attributed it to dehiscence of the diaphragm and of the pleura caused by intraperitoneal adhesions and high pneumoperitoneal pressure.

### *Mediastinal Emphysema*

Wenderoth (1954) described two cases of mediastinal emphysema during laparoscopy. Both were characterized by the

**Table 8-1.** Mortality From Laparoscopy Reported in the Literature

| Date | Author | Total Cases | Mortality No. | Mortality % | Diagnoses* |
|---|---|---|---|---|---|
| 1943 | Walker et al. | 2000 | 2 | 0.10 | Liver biopsy with hemorrhage (1)<br>Debilitated patient (1) |
| 1949 | Ruddock | 2500 | 3 | 0.12 | Liver biopsy with hemorrhage (1)<br>Spleen biopsy with hemorrhage (1)<br>Peritonitis post-laparotomy (1) |
| 1951 | Kalk and Bruhl | 2000 | 0 | 0 | |
| 1951 | Jernstrom | ? | 1 | ? | Air embolism through abdominal wall veins (1) |
| 1951 | Benedict | 914 | 5 | 0.55 | Coronary occlusion, lung abscesses (1)<br>Liver biopsy (2)<br>Tuberculous peritonitis with colon perforation (1)<br>Liver biopsy, biliary cirrhosis (1) |
| 1955 | Hartlieb | ? | 2 | ? | Pulmonary emboli (2) |
| 1955 | Rosenbaum | 800 | 0 | 0 | |

*Number in parentheses refers to number of patients.

development of an enormous emphysema on the skin of the breast and neck, causing symptoms of compression and suffocation. The air was immediately released from the abdomen and the examination terminated. X-ray photographs showed air in the mediastinum which was absorbed during the next few days, after which the patient recovered. He quotes Towbin (1951) who reported 15 cases of mediastinal emphysema in connection with pneumoperitoneum. Wenderoth suggests two explanations for the development of mediastinal emphysema; either the peritoneum splits at the weak points of the diaphragm (aortic and esophageal hiatus) or excessive intra-abdominal pressure tears the diaphragm at points of adhesions.

Rosner (1955) described four cases of mediastinal emphysema in 102 examinations and Hörmann (1955) reported two in 150 examina-

**Table 8-1.** Mortality From Laparoscopy Reported in the Literature *(Continued)*

| DATE | AUTHOR | TOTAL CASES | MORTALITY No. | MORTALITY % | DIAGNOSES* |
|---|---|---|---|---|---|
| 1956 | Wildhirt† | 350 | 1 | 0.29 | Mediastinal emphysema (8 cases reported, 7 survived) (1) |
| 1956 | Handley and Nurick | 4606 | 10 | 0.21 | Liver biopsy complications (7)<br>Peritonitis (1)<br>Bowel perforation (1)<br>Cardiac-pulmonary complication (1) |
| 1962 | Kalk and Wildhirt | 6129 | 2 | 0.03 | Liver cirrhosis, venous hemorrhage (1)<br>Cardiac decompensation (1) |
| 1965 | Frangenheim | 1850 | 0 | 0 | |
| 1965 | Frangenheim (verbal reports) | ? | 4 | ? | Air emboli (4) |
| 1968 | Vilardell et al. | 1455 | 2 | 0.13 | Liver cirrhosis, hemorrhage from abdominal wall vein (1)<br>Removal of large amount of ascitic fluid in hepatic coma (1) |

†Cited in reports, by Wenderoth (1954), Hörmann (1955), and Rosner (1955).

tions. In both cases Hörmann observed skin emphysemata in the supraclavicular areas due to high abdominal pressure; x-ray photographs showed air in the mediastinum. He ascribed the mediastinal emphysema to hiatus hernia. One of Rosner's cases was subjected to autopsy; the patient suffering from liver metastases developed emphysema in the jugular and cervical areas during liver biopsy. X-ray examination showed the presence of air in the mediastinum. After a few days both internal and external emphysemas were absorbed, but the patient subsequently died from hepatic coma.

Wildhirt (1956) reported that he had not observed a single case of mediastinal emphysema in 5000 examinations.

Steinberg (1956) reported one case of mediastinal emphysema

with accompanying emphysema of the neck among 150 examinations. He theorized that under certain circumstances air passes from the abdominal cavity into the thoracic cavity in the region of the sternocostal fibrous trigone, that is, where the aorta, the vena cava, and the esophagus enter.

Wittman (1966) observed abdominal wall emphysema in a few cases. This is probably due to sudden changes in abdominal wall pressure brought about by straining and vomiting.

When reporting mediastinal emphysema most authors describe simultaneous subcutaneous emphysema extending to the skin of the neck. Therefore, air could travel subcutaneously along the abdomen and the thorax to the neck and from there through the deep fascia of the neck to the mediastinum.

Frangenheim (1965) stated that the majority of complications arises when the pneumoperitoneum needle is inserted to the right of and superior to the umbilicus, resulting in accidental puncture into the hepatic vein, or when the needle is inserted midway between the umbilicus and the left anterior superior iliac spine, with accidental puncture of the iliac artery. Frangenheim chooses the inferior margin of the umbilicus in the midline as the best site for both needle and trochar. He lifts the abdominal wall with the left hand, and the sharp tip of the needle is pushed through to the peritoneum. This permits insertion of the needle at a narrow angle, almost parallel to the abdominal wall. The development of emphysema is prevented by keeping the needle in motion during insufflation. If the tip of the needle enters the omentum, mesentery, or the preperitoneal space, this is corrected by judicious reinsertion. Equal distribution of gas within and distention of the peritoneal cavity is checked by repeated percussion. Liver dullness must disappear.

### *Cardiac Arrest*

Friedberg (1966) defines cardiac arrest as the sudden stoppage of the heart and circulation following cardiac ventricular standstill or ventricular fibrillation. Its frequency in the course of surgery has been reported by Glenn (1953) as one case in 3673, by Stephenson et al. (1953) as one in 2382, and by West (1954) as one in 1200 cases. It may occur prior to the introduction of the pneumoperitoneum, during induction of anesthesia, or during endotracheal intubation. It is induced by cardiac anoxia from any cause. Should cardiac arrest occur, the anesthetist immediately stops all anesthetic agents and gases except oxygen. Establishment of an adequate airway or intubation is essential. External massage should be instituted at once. In the operating room, internal open massage may be resorted to if external massage proves ineffectual. The technique of transthoracic massage is well presented in Bailey (1967).

A gynecologist working in a small community hospital in Indiana recently called to report a case of cardiac arrest that occurred while he was inducing a pneumoperitoneum prior to laparoscopy. The indication for this procedure was unexplained pelvic pain. The anesthesia was sodium thiopental* and nitrous oxide, without intubation. The Verres needle was inserted through the right lower quadrant, and the carbon dioxide gas introduced under pressure did not exceed 40 mm. of mercury. When the anesthetist announced that there was no blood pressure, pulse, or heartbeat detectable, closed cardiac massage was performed. A portable x-ray was obtained, and when the film was subsequently viewed, it showed a pneumomediastinum and bilateral pneumothorax. Although cardiac function was reestablished, the patient died within 48 hours. Postmortem examination revealed that the needle had perforated the posterior parietal peritoneum into the fascial spaces surrounding the iliac vessels. Apparently the carbon dioxide gas found easy access upwards to induce a massive pneumomediastinum and pneumothorax.

Let us examine the technique employed in this case to determine whether there are safeguards that could have prevented the tragic outcome. Although we personally do not use the right lower quadrant for inserting the Verres needle, it is considered an acceptable site, especially by gastroenterologists attempting to avoid an enlarged liver. The junction of the outer and middle thirds of a line from the umbilicus to the anterior superior iliac spine is approved also as a site for paracentesis. Most gynecologists use the periumbilical area, although some insert a needle 5 cm. below the umbilicus in the midline. Palmer employs the left infracostal area where the peritoneum is fixed. Stein prefers a site 1 cm. above and to the left of the umbilicus. Also, a point at the level of the umbilicus in the mammary line may be used should laparotomy scars interfere with selection of another site.

Wittman suggests various tests to make certain that the needle is in the free peritoneal cavity, such as gently moving the needle to determine whether the point touches an abdominal organ. In the Indiana case cited above, the tip of the needle must have been fixed. If it had been withdrawn a centimeter or two it would have entered the free peritoneal cavity. It is further suggested that the needle be moved constantly while creating the pneumoperitoneum to prevent accumulations of gas in the omentum, for example. We routinely point the needle toward the pelvic concavity.

When the needle is in the peritoneal cavity, it is kept parallel to the abdominal wall, which has been elevated manually during the introduction of gas. Wittman (1966) suggests injecting 20 to 40 ml. of air by syringe through the pneumoperitoneum needle as a final

*Pentothal, sodium, Abbott Laboratories, North Chicago, Ill.

check prior to inducing the pneumoperitoneum. If the end of the needle is in the abdominal wall, subcutaneous emphysema is created. Any minor air embolism which may have been created by this small amount of air (20 to 40 ml.) could be recognized by observing the patient for a minute or two. Wittman believes that there is no greater risk in using air, although carbon dioxide is preferred in gynecologic laparoscopy.

We use either Innovar plus local anesthesia or general anesthesia with intubation. For general anesthesia we prefer fluothane rather than nitrous oxide gas. The use of intubation provides the anesthetist with complete control over pulmonary ventilation.

Unfortunately, in the tragic Indiana case just described the diagnosis of pneumomediastinum and pneumothorax was not made immediately, although a portable chest film had been obtained. Had this diagnosis been made, immediate mediastinal and chest needling might have had most dramatic beneficial effects. Had open cardiac massage been performed in this case, a life might have been saved.

As in any surgical technique, complications may occur. Statistically, they are extremely rare and are chiefly due to inexperience. The laparoscopist must pay attention to the most minute detail, especially when inducing the pneumoperitoneum. In the literature most of the serious complications have occurred during upper abdominal laparoscopy in seriously ill patients. In gynecologic laparoscopy the patient is usually young and relatively healthy. The laparoscopist must be aware of the possibility of complications and be alert enough to avoid them.

*Chapter Nine*

# INTERVAL TUBAL STERILIZATION VIA LAPAROSCOPY


MELVIN R. COHEN, M.D.
MARSHALL BENNETT TAYLOR, M.D.*
MARTIN B. KASS, M.D.*


After diagnostic proficiency with laparoscopy is attained, certain surgical procedures such as tubal sterilization may be easily performed. Anderson, in a 1937 report concerning new instruments, stated that tubal sterilization by endothermic coagulation could be performed via peritoneoscopy. Power and Barnes (1941) described a method of tubal sterilization in association with laparoscopy in which they cauterized the cornual portion of each tube and a segment some 3 to 5 cm. distally. There appears to have been a hiatus of interest in sterilization associated with laparoscopy until its recent reintroduction by Palmer (1963), Frangenheim (1964), and Steptoe (1967). Steptoe described cauterizing the tube at two points and then dividing it midway between the cauterized areas. Thus each tube is grasped at three points. We have felt it necessary to modify this method to satisfy two objectives: (1) to avoid the occasional bleeding encountered, and (2) to obtain segments of the uterine tubes for histological examination and documentation.

Our series consists of 50 interval tubal sterilizations performed during laparoscopy. Our modifications basically involve coagulating,


*The Department of Obstetrics and Gynecology, Michael Reese Hospital and Medical Center, The Fertility Institute, Chicago, Illinois

dividing, and retrieving a section of tissue, all by grasping each tube just once.

## MATERIALS AND METHODS

Nonexplosive general anesthesia with endotracheal intubation or local skin anesthesia with neuroleptanalgesia (see Chapter 4) is used. The state of neuroleptanalgesia is induced by a narcotic (fentanyl[*]) combined with a major tranquilizer (droperidol[†]) injected intravenously. The perineum, vagina, and abdomen are prepared with a nonflammable antiseptic solution such as povidone iodine.[‡] The indifferent electrode of the Bovie electrosurgical unit is placed in contact with the lumbosacral region of the patient. The patient's bladder is emptied and bimanual examination performed. A self-retaining tubal patency cannula is then inserted into the cervical canal. A pneumoperitoneum is created using carbon dioxide gas injected at a flow of one liter per minute to distend the abdomen wall. The patient is then placed at a 30° to 35° Trendelenburg position, and laparoscopy is performed in the usual manner.

Inspection is made of the pelvic organs. If necessary, the uterus may be moved by means of the intra-uterine cannula. The lower abdomen is then transilluminated by holding the laparoscope against the anterior peritoneum to allow selection of an avascular area in the right lower quadrant. At a point about 6 cm. lateral to the midline

*Sublimaze, McNeil Laboratories, Fort Washington, Pa.
†Inapsine (Sublimaze with Inapsine is available commercially as Innovar)
‡Betadine, Purdue Frederick Co., Yonkers, N.Y.

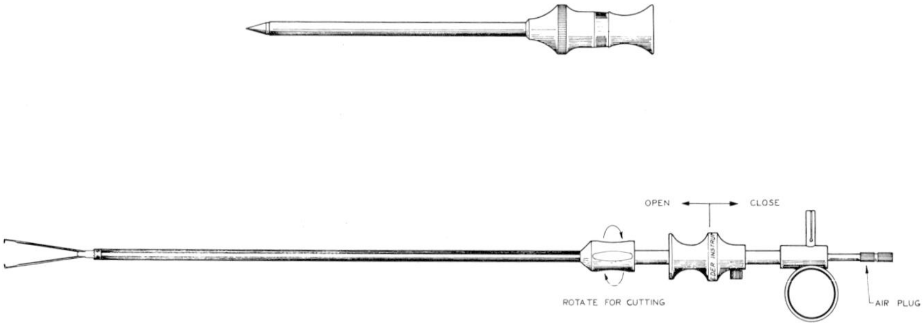


Figure 9–1. Cohen-Eder biopsy tong, a modification of the Palmer biopsy drill forceps. *Above*, 6 mm. conical trochar and sleeve without valve. *Below*, biopsy tong with 2.5 mm. interlumen diameter.

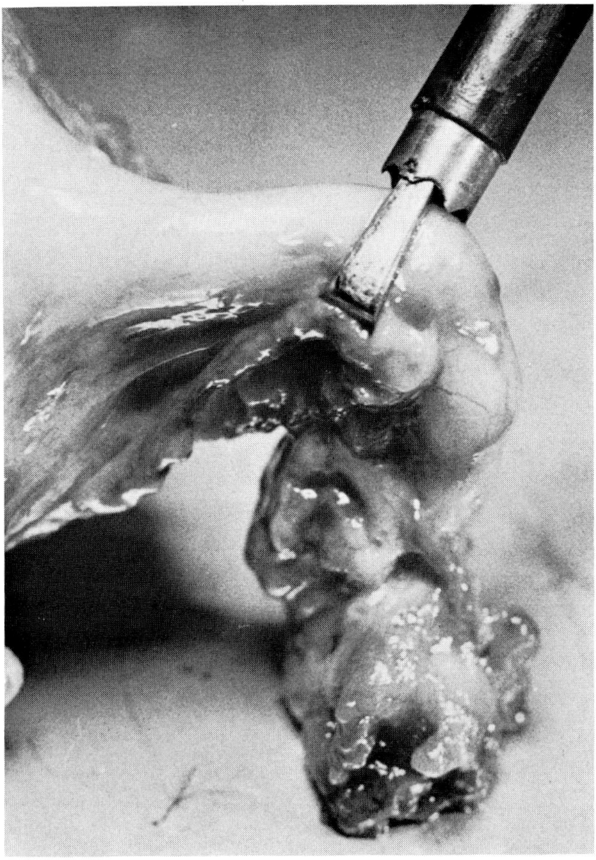

*Figure* 9–2. Demonstration of Cohen-Eder biopsy tong grasping tube of extirpated specimen, preparatory to cautery excision. Note cylindrical cutting drill in place.

and 6 cm. above the inguinal ligament, a small stab wound is made. A 6-mm. cannula, to accommodate the Palmer biopsy forceps* or its modification, the Cohen-Eder biopsy tong† (Fig. 9–1), with its trochar, is introduced into the peritoneal cavity. Introduction of the forceps through this cannula permits the surgeon to grasp the uterine tube easily. The laparoscopic headclamp (Taylor, 1969) frees the operator's hands for more efficient control of the forceps.

One tube is grasped with the forceps at a point about 2 cm. from the cornu and held with gentle traction (Fig. 9–2). Under direct vision, and with care that the tip of the forceps is not in contact with any other tissue, a moderate wave of cutting current at 30 per cent

*Drapier, S.A., Paris, France
†Eder Instrument Company, Chicago, Ill.

intensity is applied. This is sustained and the tube is seen to blanch radially from the tip of the forceps. When a section of tube 1 cm. on either side of the tip has been coagulated, the current is discontinued. This usually requires four to six seconds, but the end point is the visible radial coagulation, not the time needed. Without removing the forceps tip, the sawtoothed outer cannula is then screwed downward. As it cuts through the tube, the cutting current is again momentarily applied until the cannula disengages from its track. By holding the sawtoothed cannula in place and withdrawing the forceps, the surgeon is able to remove the severed section of tube. In a similar manner the opposite tube is grasped, coagulated, severed, and a section excised and retrieved. The separated severed ends of each tube must be visualized (and hemostasis verified) before the procedure is considered complete. The section of tube obtained, although evidencing signs of the coagulation, can be identified histologically (Fig. 9–3). Twenty-four hours later the skin clips are removed from the two miniature incisions and the patient is discharged. She may return to full activity immediately.

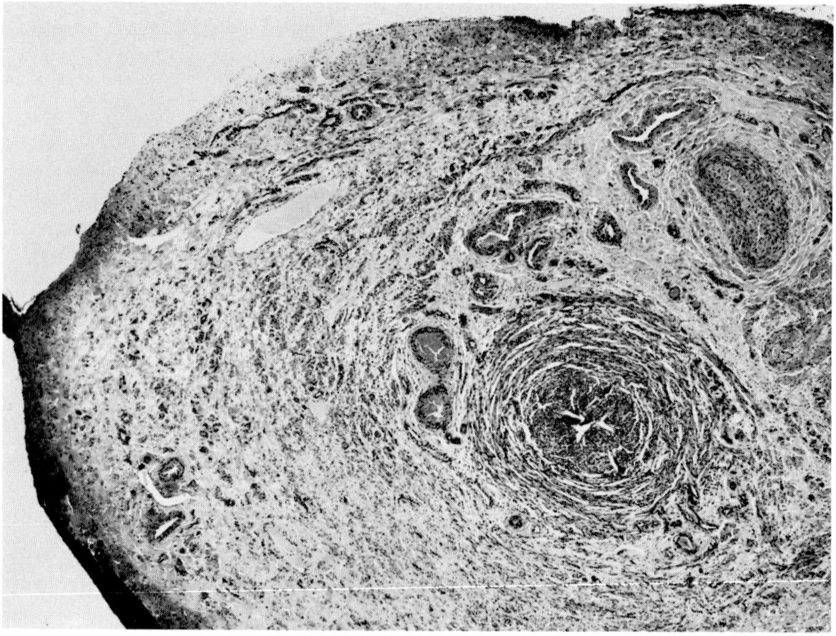

*Figure 9–3.* Histologic evidence of cautery excision of fallopian tube. × 7. Good preservation of cellular detail is shown despite cauterization of distal portions of resected segment.

**Table 9–1.** Indications for Laparoscopic Interval Sterilization by Age Group

| | NUMBER OF CASES | | |
|---|---|---|---|
| INDICATIONS | *20-29 Years* | *30-39 Years* | *Over 40 Years* |
| Multiparity | 12 | 25 | 3 |
| Diabetes | – | 1 | – |
| Mental retardation | 2 | 1 | – |
| Rh sensitization | – | 1 | – |
| Hypertension | 1 | 1 | – |
| Cardiac disease | – | 1 | – |
| Previous cesarean section | – | 1 | – |
| Multiple sclerosis with thrombophlebitis | – | 1 | – |
| Total | 15 | 32 | 3 |

## RESULTS

In the period from October, 1967, through February, 1969, 50 interval sterilizations were performed at Michael Reese Hospital by the method just described. The patients ranged in age from 20 to 41 years with an average of 31.5 years. The indications, grouped by age, are shown in Table 9–1. When the indication was multiparity, the average number of children was 5.7.

Nine patients had hysterograms from two to six months after surgery. Nine additional patients underwent repeat laparoscopy. In all cases tubal occlusion was verified. In one of our patients hysterosalpingography demonstrated partial tubal patency on one side. However, at repeat laparoscopy, with pertubation of an indigo carmine solution, both tubes were found to be completely occluded. It is known that this hysterogram was performed under high pressure, and we believe that this created a temporary opening in the proximal tube. There have been no pregnancies in this group of patients, now with an average follow-up period of ten months. There have not been any complications either immediately postoperatively or during the follow-up period.

## COMMENT

Operative interruption of the uterine tubes is firmly established in our armamentarium of sterilization techniques. Most would agree that the immediate postpartum period represents the optimal time for such a procedure because the tubes are most accessible at this time and a subsequent conception, occurring before a delayed procedure can be done, may be averted. Nonetheless, postpartum surgery must be delayed occasionally for such interdicting conditions as anemia, infection, or toxemia. Medical indications may subsequently arise, and patients may with justification seek sterilization at a later date.

Although Anderson (1937) and Power and Barnes (1941) suggested a method of sterilization in association with laparoscopy, they did not report any cases or results. More recently Palmer (1963) reported his results on 10 patients as did Frangenheim in 1964 with 17 patients. Steptoe (1965), utilizing the instrument of Palmer, demonstrated this very simple, safe, and effective technique in a large series of patients in England. He has since reported (Steptoe, 1969) that 310 patients have been treated in the two-year period beginning January 1, 1966, by a technique of diathermy division of the tubes at laparoscopy.

In a review of 29,496 tubal sterilizations by the classic abdominal or vaginal route, Garb (1957) reported an overall failure rate of 0.71 per cent. It should be noted that the preponderance of these procedures were performed in the immediate postpartum period. Steptoe (1969) reports one failure in 310 laparoscopic sterilizations, a failure rate of 0.3 per cent. This single failure was a tubal ectopic pregnancy. We have observed no failures in our 50 cases to date.

Compared to the classic methods of interval sterilization via laparotomy or colpotomy, operative laparoscopy appears to offer decided advantages:

1. The patient is only briefly hospitalized.
2. She undergoes a short general or local anesthesia.
3. There is little or no postoperative discomfort.
4. The miniature incisions leave no unsightly scars.
5. Good visualization of all the pelvic organs can be obtained while performing this procedure.

In our opinion, the results of sterilization in conjunction with laparoscopy are comparable to, if not better than, the classic methods.

*Chapter Ten*

# OVARIAN BIOPSY AND ANCILLARY TECHNIQUES

To perform surgical procedures by way of the laparoscope, such as lysis of adhesions, ovarian biopsy, or aspiration of ovarian cysts, the operating peritoneoscope, or laparoscope (Fig. 10–1), is used, or a second trochar and cannula is inserted through the lower abdominal wall (Fig. 10–2). A manipulative probe, various cautery tips, grasping forceps, a suction cannula, and scissors may be inserted through one of these instruments (Figs. 10–3 and 10–4), and a surgical diathermy cord can be attached to permit lysis of fine adhesions or cautery under direct vision. I have previously described my technique of ovarian needle biopsy via peritoneoscopy (Cohen, 1968*b*).

Problems in human reproduction could be solved more easily if the ovary were as accessible to biopsy as the endometrium. The ovary, because of its pedicle, is a very mobile pelvic organ. It is essential that biopsy of this "moving target" be relatively bloodless and atraumatic.

With the establishment of an adequate pneumoperitoneum under pressure, a 6 mm. cannula with trochar may be safely inserted through the lower abdomen. The trochar is removed and the Palmer drill biopsy forceps (Fig. 10–5) or the Cohen-Eder biopsy tong (Fig. 9–1) is introduced. The Cohen-Eder biopsy tong has two fingerlike prongs which enable the surgeon to grasp each ovary without trauma. The Palmer and Cohen-Eder instruments are fitted with their own biopsy mechanism, activated by surgical diathermy. However, we have found that a cautery technique destroys too much

*Text continues on page 62*

**Fiber Light Jacobs-Palmer Operating Peritoneoscope**

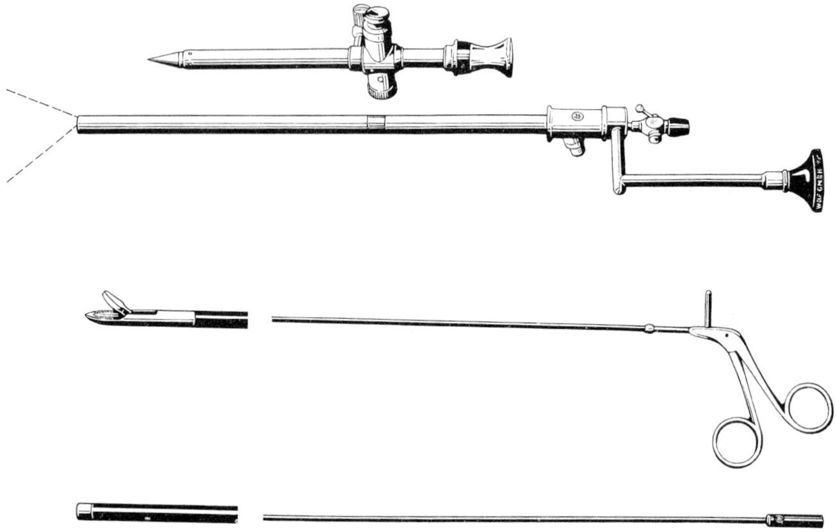

*Figure 10–1.* Fiber light Jacobs-Palmer operating peritoneoscope (laparoscope). Manufactured by Richard Wolf, Knittlingen, West Germany; distributed by Eder Instrument Company, Chicago, Ill.

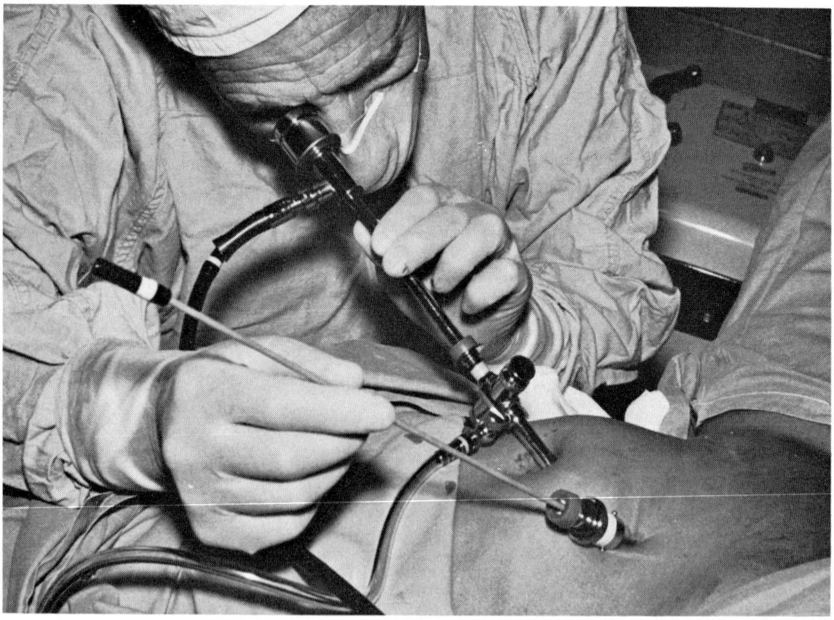

*Figure 10–2.* Ancillary surgical procedure through separate cannula, here held in the surgeon's right hand.

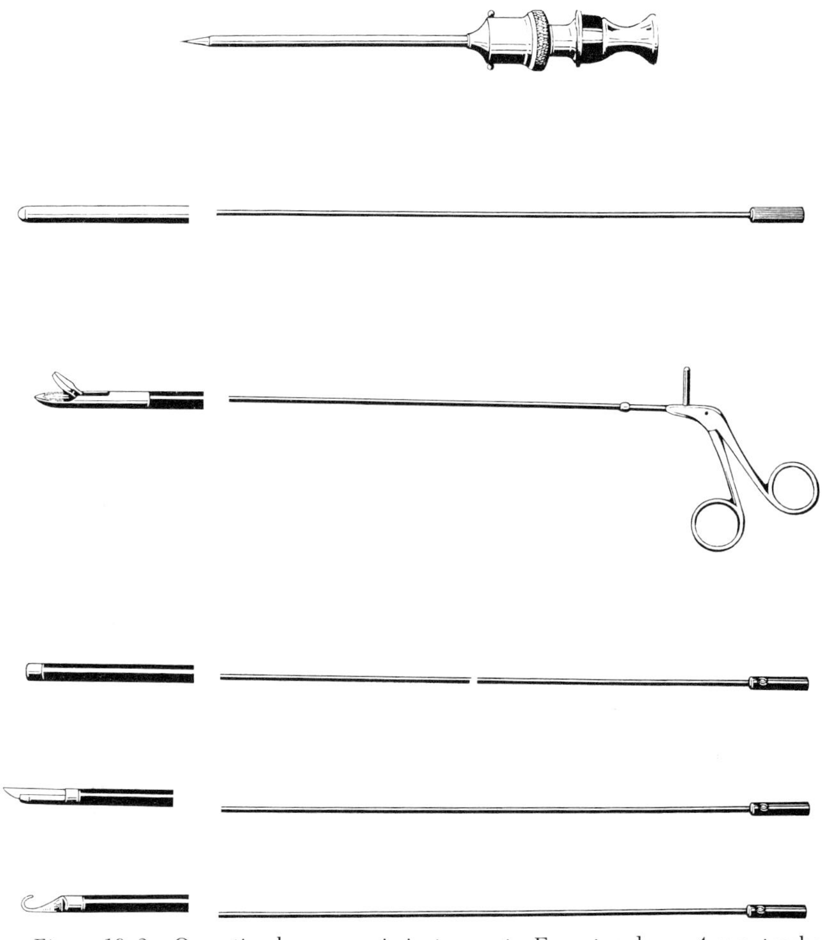

*Figure 10–3.* Operative laparoscopic instruments. From top down: 4 mm. trochar and sleeve, manipulative probe, biopsy forceps, cautery probe, cautery knife, and cautery hook.

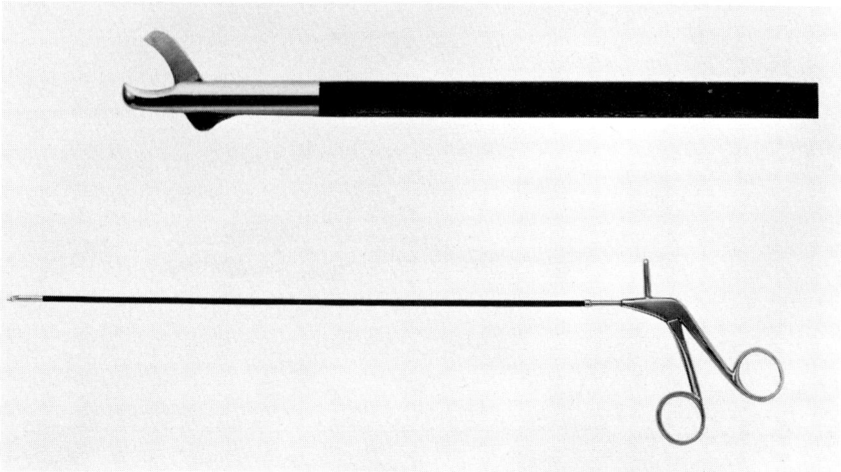

*Figure 10–4.* Insulated scissors with attachment for surgical diathermy cord. This may be inserted through a 4 mm. trochar and sleeve.

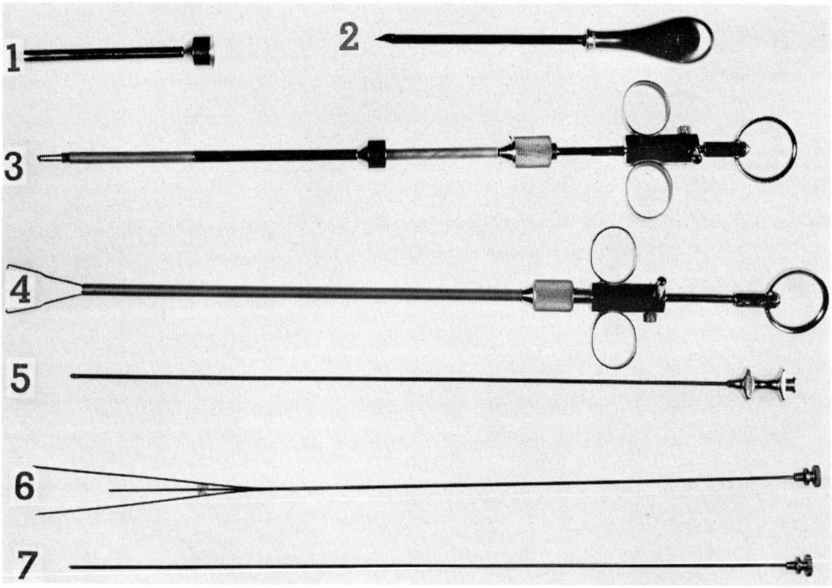


*Figure 10–5.* Ovarian biopsy instruments: (*1*) cannula; (*2*) trochar; (*3*) Palmer forceps inserted through cannula in closed position; (*4*) Palmer forceps with jaws expanded; (*5*) Franklin Silverman needle sleeve; (*6*) Franklin Silverman needle biopsy stylet with prongs separated; and (*7*) Franklin Silverman needle obdurator. (From Cohen, M. R. [1968*b*]: Ovarian biopsy via peritoneoscopy. J. Reprod. Med. *1*:436.)

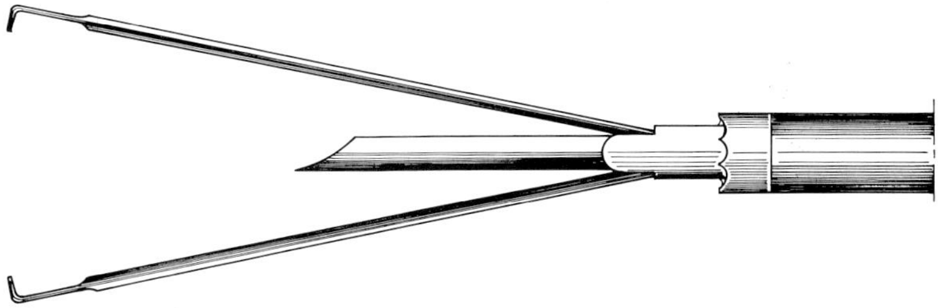

*Figure 10–6.* Detail of Cohen-Eder biopsy tong with needle protruding through channel which allows insertion of biopsy needles or suction tubes up to 2.5 mm.

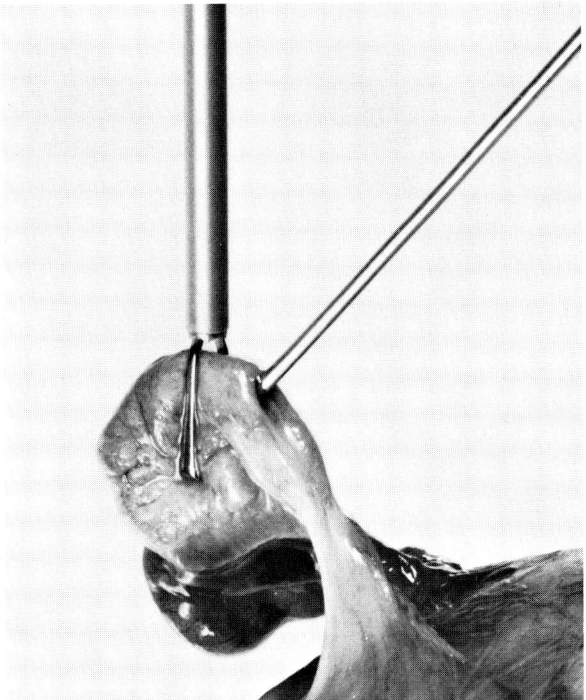

*Figure 10–7.* Ovarian biopsy technique on extirpated surgical specimen. Cohen-Eder biopsy tong holds ovary while needle biopsy is being obtained. (From Cohen, M. R. [1968*b*]: Ovarian biopsy via peritoneoscopy. J. Reprod. Med. *1*:436.)

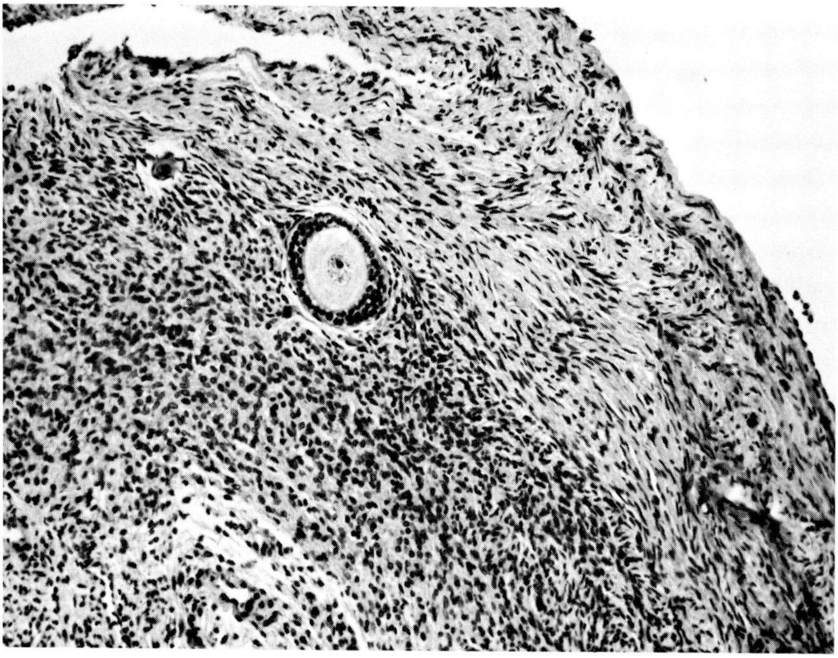

*Figure 10–8.* Photomicrograph of biopsy obtained from ovary at laparoscopy. × 200.

tissue. Hence, the instrument is used only to grasp and steady the ovary.

While the ovary is held, a Franklin Silverman needle,* 33 cm. in length (Fig. 10–5), is inserted through the capsule of the ovary and a sliver of tissue is obtained. The Cohen-Eder biopsy tong has a channel that accommodates the biopsy needle (Fig. 10–6) and guides it to the area of biopsy. This procedure may be repeated to obtain biopsies in other areas of the ovary. It is then possible to grasp the other ovary and obtain one or several additional biopsies. The areas of puncture usually do not bleed. Immediately after biopsies are obtained, the ovary appears relatively intact. Figure 10–7 illustrates the technique on a surgically extirpated ovary. The specimen obtained in this manner (Fig. 10–8) shows good histologic preservation and is useful for most diagnostic purposes.

We have found this technique especially useful in patients with an ovulatory amenorrhea prior to therapy with HMG-HCG or clomiphene citrate. The presence of primordial follicles in ovarian biopsies obtained in these cases is a good prognostic finding.

*V. Mueller and Company, Chicago, Illinois

*Chapter Eleven*

# LAPAROSCOPIC PHOTOGRAPHY

The problems inherent in endoscopic photography have been resolved with the use of luminous optics to transmit more light through the endoscope, a more powerful source of "cold light," the use of electronic flash equipment, and fast color film. The new 1000 watt General Electric lamp, incorporated in both the American Cystoscope and the Eder fiber optic power supplies, provides good illumination for 16 mm. movies with Ektachrome daylight film, ASA rating 160. We have used the Beaulieu 16 mm. electric drive camera (Fig. 11–1) at a speed of 40 frames per second with a 25 mm. lens adapted to the Richard Wolf 10 mm. 135° photographic laparoscope and to the Richard Wolf 8 mm. diagnostic laparoscope. Still color photographs of excellent quality may be obtained with these laparoscopes (Fig. 11–2); the power supply and film type are the same as for cinematography, and a single lens reflex camera is used with special adapters.

For more professional color transparencies we recommend the Wolf electronic flash (strobe) (Fig. 11–3). This technique is more complicated, however. A 10 mm. trochar and cannula is inserted through the abdominal wall. The trochar is removed, and the cannula will then accommodate a sleeve containing a 6 volt incandescent lamp, which provides sufficient light for adequate pelvic and abdominal visualization. The sleeve will accommodate the laparoscope, which has a 135° optic, and a miniaturized electronic flash bulb activated by way of an insulated cord from the power supply. The photo-laparoscope is then locked securely in place inside the sleeve.

It is also possible to use a fiber optic sleeve. This fiber optic

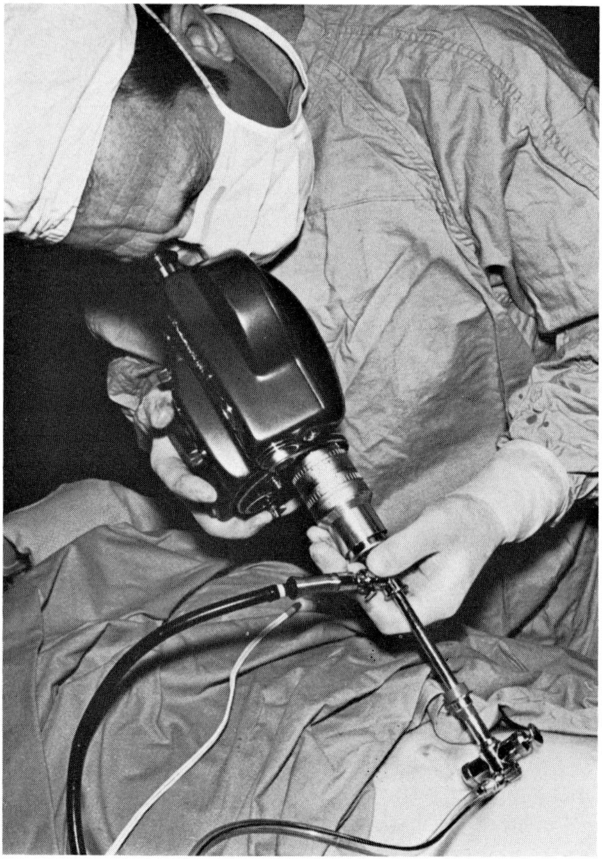

*Figure 11–1.* Cinematography with Beaulieu 16 mm. camera adapted to Wolf 10 mm. laparascope.

sleeve is a millimeter larger than the incandescent sleeve, and hence a larger trochar and cannula must be used. Further, the fiber optic sleeve contains a rather small bundle for transmitting light so that we have found it necessary to use a power source which incorporates the 1000 watt General Electric photographic lamp. My preference is the incandescent sleeve, and although the illumination from such a bulb is not color corrected for daylight film, the strobe, or electronic flash, completely dominates this light. We have not had any disappointments in the color quality of the transparencies.

There is a theoretical objection to inserting an optical instrument with electronic flash bulb into the body cavity. Inasmuch as the voltage is very high (800 volts) and even though the amperage is extremely low, this bulb must be well insulated. The bulb is protected by a metal tip which has a transparent plastic window cemented into its metal housing. Should there be any defect in the

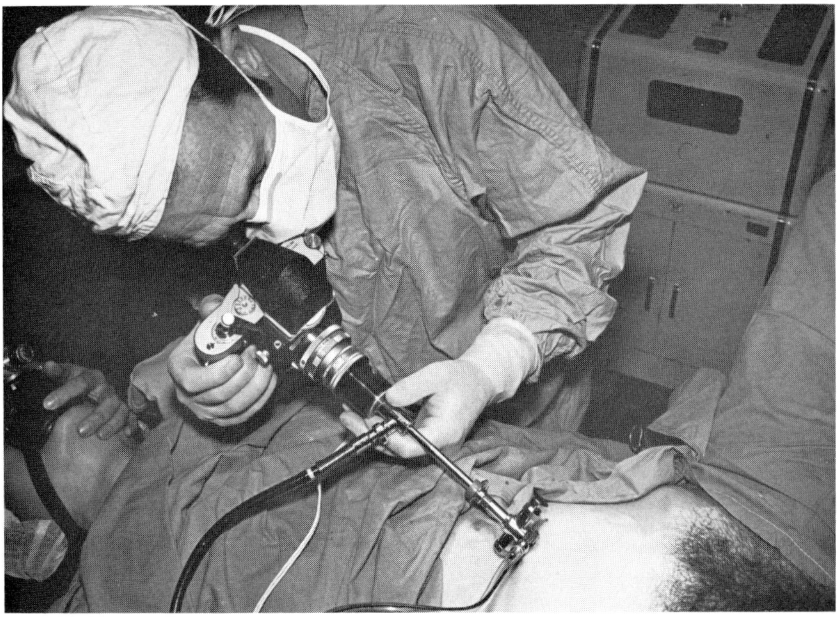

*Figure 11–2.* Still photography with Leicaflex camera adapted to Wolf 10 mm. laparoscope.

plastic cement, it is possible for moisture to penetrate the metal housing of this bulb. The housing containing the bulb is screwed into the laparoscope. The threads at this connection should be lubricated with the special grease supplied with the laparoscope.

Recently, while photographing at operation, I noted that a mild electrical shock was sustained by one of my patients under general anesthesia. This transient shock had no harmful effects. The instruments were removed, and careful inspection revealed a minute defect in the plastic cement. The plastic window was resealed and I have had no trouble since. When instruments are gas sterilized, there is little chance for moisture to seep into the bulb housing or plastic window. However, when more than one laparoscopy is performed, it is necessary to cold sterilize the instruments, and therefore it is essential to carefully inspect the Wolf photo-laparoscope prior to use.

Any single lens reflex camera with an electronic flash shutter attachment may be adapted to the laparoscope. We have used a Leicaflex camera with a 90 mm. lens and the Olympus Pen F camera with a 75 mm. lens. A special power transformer supplies the required voltage with three settings: closeup, midrange, and panoramic. Excellent photographs, measuring 15 mm. in diameter, have been obtained with Ektachrome X daylight film, ASA rating 64. (See Chapter 17.)

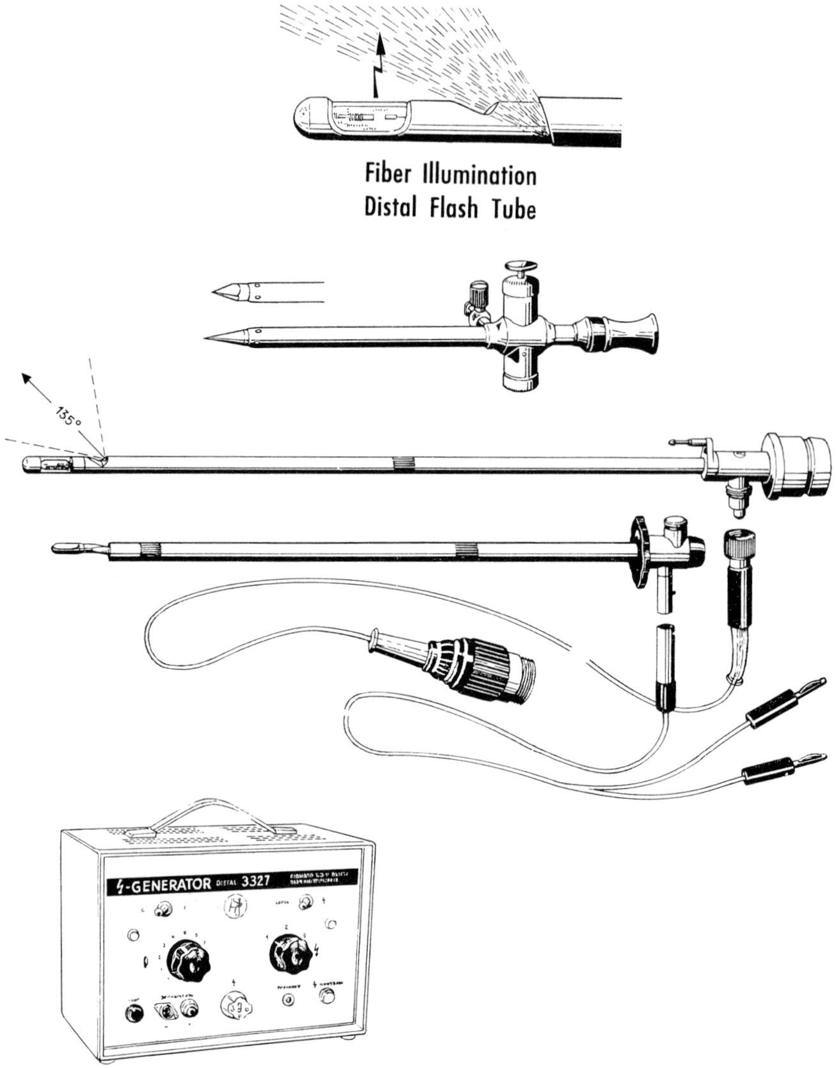


*Figure 11–3.* Flash laparoscope, manufactured by Richard Wolf, Knittlingen, West Germany; distributed by AGA Corporation, Secaucus, N.J. and Eder Instrument Company, Chicago, Ill. From top down: fiber optic illumination in sleeve, with detail of distal flash bulb; cannula and trochar with the two types of perforators; flash laparoscope with 135° lens; sleeve containing 6 volt incandescent bulb; flash and incandescent cord; power supply for incandescent lamp and electronic flash.

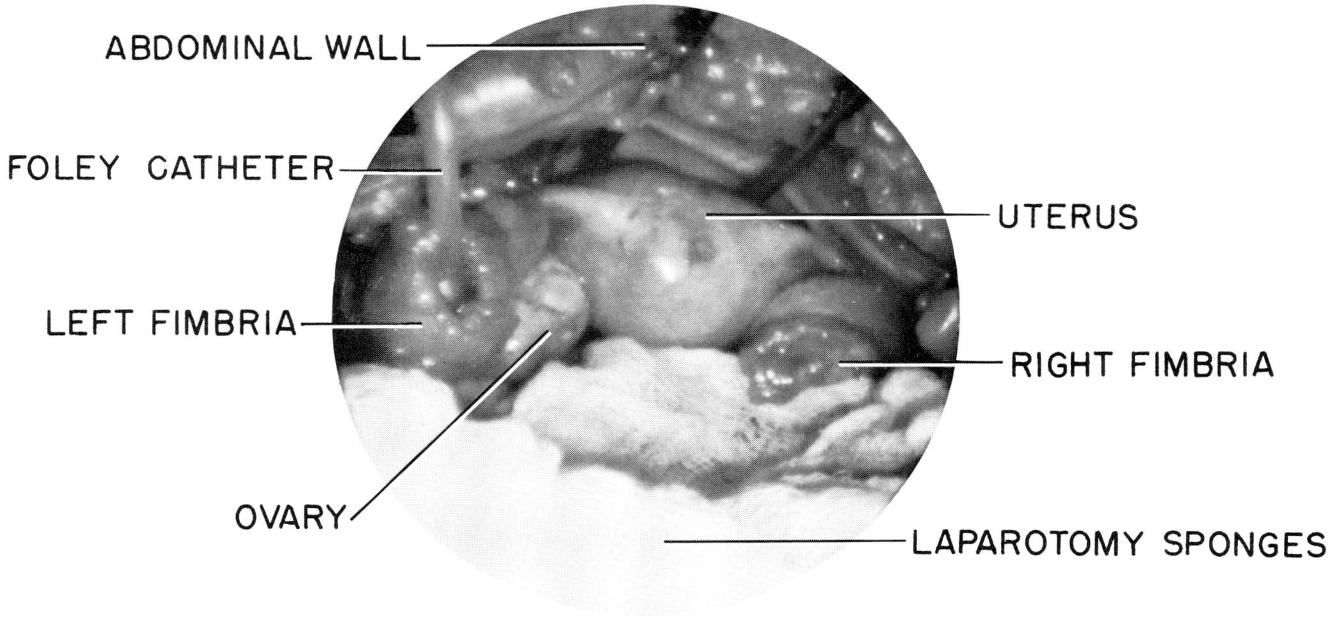


*Figure 11–4.* Example of photograph obtained at laparotomy showing reconstructed right fimbria completed and left fimbria being reconstructed with a #8 pediatric Foley catheter. Demonstration of author's technique for tuboplasty in hydrosalpinx.

I personally use the Wolf photo-laparoscope for all routine cases—one never knows when photography may be desired. Furthermore, this instrument is suitable for photography in vivo during laparotomy to document operative technique and findings (Fig. 11-4).

The Menghini-Wildhirt peritoneoscope* has an external strobe attachment which is ingeniously devised, but which I have found rather cumbersome. The peritoneoscope itself consists of a metal housing that contains a channel for an optic unit consisting of a quartz rod for transmission of fiber optic light, as well as the surge of light induced by the electronic flash, and a channel for ancillary surgical techniques, including biopsy and so forth. This apparatus is quite complicated and cannot be recommended for the novice, although the advantage of having an external electronic flash rather than one incorporated in the distal end of the laparoscope within the body cavity is obvious. The Menghini-Wildhirt scope is equipped with a power supply for synchronized flash. Although I was able to utilize this instrument in vitro and obtained excellent color transparencies on excised surgical specimens, I was not successful in obtaining satisfactory transparencies during laparoscopy. The photographs in the atlas (Chapter 17) were taken with the Wolf electronic flash (strobe) laparoscope.

---

*Storz Instrument Company, St. Louis, Mo.

*Chapter Twelve*

# CULDOSCOPY AND CULDOSCOPIC PHOTOGRAPHY

## CULDOSCOPY

Decker, the "father of culdoscopy," was originally a peritoneoscopist. In 1944, he and Cherry described an easy method for inducing a pneumoperitoneum spontaneously by cul-de-sac puncture with the patient in knee-chest position. Decker showed that an endoscopic instrument could be introduced safely through the vagina for excellent visualization of the intrapelvic viscera. This procedure, which he called culdoscopy, may be performed in the clinic or outpatient department under local anesthesia, thereby deleting the limiting requirements of anesthesiologist, operating room facilities, and personnel.

### *Indications*

These are similar to the indications for laparoscopy. The procedure is indicated whenever other methods of examination are insufficient to establish a diagnosis. It is especially useful in unexplained pelvic pain and suspected ectopic pregnancy. It is invaluable in the case of an infertile female when the standard tests are inconclusive and when obscure pelvic pathologic conditions are suspected. To quote Decker (1967): "Culdoscopy is not intended to confirm the obvious. Large pelvic tumors or masses are best treated by laparotomy."

### *Contraindications*

Contraindications for culdoscopy are as follows:

1. Vaginitis; acute cervicitis.
2. Vaginal atresia.
3. The patient's inability to assume the knee-chest position due to cardiac or respiratory difficulties.
4. The absence of a free cul-de-sac due to a fixed retroversion or cul-de-sac mass. If puncture into a free cul-de-sac does not occur, the procedure cannot be performed.
5. Acute pelvic inflammatory disease.
6. Ruptured ectopic pregnancy.
7. Age per se is no contraindication, although children and the very old are usually poor subjects for this technique.

### *Technique*

Culdoscopy is a procedure that requires sterile precautions. The following outlined procedure, modified from Decker (1967), represents that presently employed at Michael Reese Hospital.

1. Preparation of patient.
   (a) The genitalia need not be shaven.
   (b) A cleansing enema is given.
   (c) Premedication consists of a narcotic, such as meperidine, 100 mg., prochlorperazine,* 10 mg. (an antiemetic tranquilizing drug), plus scopolamine, not to exceed 0.4 mg. intramuscularly one hour prior to the procedure. This basal analgesia may be augmented by additional intravenous narcotics at the time of the procedure. Premedication with meperidine, 100 mg., plus hydroxyzine hydrochloride,† 50 mg. intravenously, is routine for outpatient culdoscopies.
2. Position of patient.
   The patient is placed on an ordinary operating room table in knee-chest position. She is kept in this position by means of shoulder braces. A soft, 4-inch thick pad supports the breasts and shoulders and prevents angulation of the neck. The foot of the table is released, permitting the legs of the patient to project halfway from the table. We find the use of the Decker knee rest unnecessary. Upright leg holders are frequently used to prevent lateral flexion of the patient while in knee-chest position.

---

*Compazine, Smith Kline and French Laboratories, Philadelphia, Pa.
†Vistaril, Pfizer Laboratories, New York, N.Y.

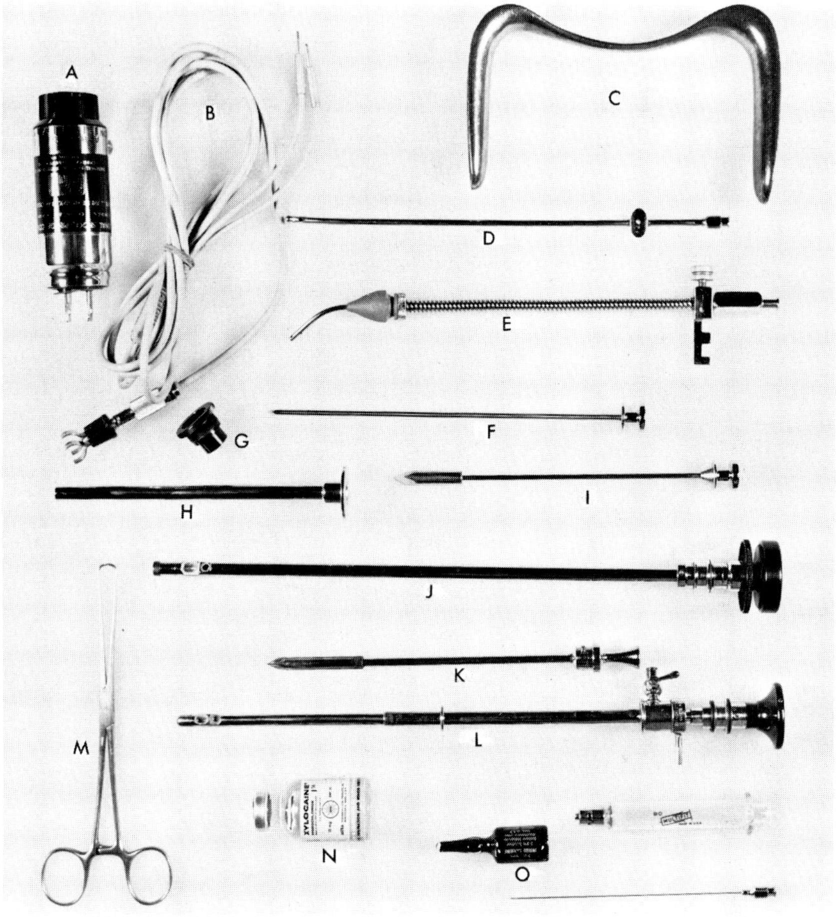


*Figure 12–1.* Basic equipment for culdoscopy, tubal patency, and endometrial biopsy: (*A*) voltage transformer; (*B*) light cord; (*C*) Sims speculum; (*D*) endometrial biopsy curette; (*E*) patency cannula (Cohen); (*F*) small Clyman trochar for cul-de-sac identification; (*G*) movie adapter; (*H*) Clyman cannula; (*I*) Clyman trochar; (*J*) Clyman pan-culdoscope; (*K*) Decker trochar; (*L*) Decker culdoscope in cannula; (*M*) tenaculum, short single-toothed; (*N*) Xylocaine hydrochloride solution; and (*O*) indigo carmine ampule. (From Cohen, M. R. [1964]: Culdoscopy. *In* Williams, W. W.: Sterility: The Diagnostic Survey of the Infertile Couple, Ed. 4. W. W. Williams, Springfield, Mass.

3. Preparation of genitalia and draping of patient.
   (a) The vulva and vagina are prepared with an antibacterial skin cleanser.*
   (b) The patient is draped with a single laparotomy sheet.
4. Instrumentation and anesthesia (Figs. 12–1 and 12–2). Although caudal or saddle block anesthesia may be used, it is our practice to perform this procedure under local anesthesia.
   (a) A Sims speculum is introduced into the vagina, and the rectum is retracted upward.
   (b) The posterior lip of the cervix is grasped with a single-toothed tenaculum forceps and the uterosacral ligaments identified.
   (c) The vaginal mucosa between the ligaments, the deeper structures, and the peritoneum of the cul-de-sac are infiltrated with mepivacaine hydrochloride** or a lidocaine† 1% solution. Less than 3 cc. of solution are injected into the submucosa to prevent distortion of tissue relationships and separation of mucosa from the peritoneum. If dilatation of the cervix and/or curettage is to be performed, local anesthesia is injected bilaterally into each uterosacral and cardinal ligament.
   (d) Preparation for tubal patency: The uterine canal is sounded and the cervix dilated to #4½ French. A 10-gauge Foley catheter is inserted through the cervix, and

*e.g., pHisoHex. Winthrop Laboratories, New York, N.Y., or Betadine, Purdue Frederick Company, Yonkers, N.Y.

**Carbocaine, Winthrop Laboratories, New York, N.Y.

†Xylocaine, Astra Products, Inc., Worcester, Mass.

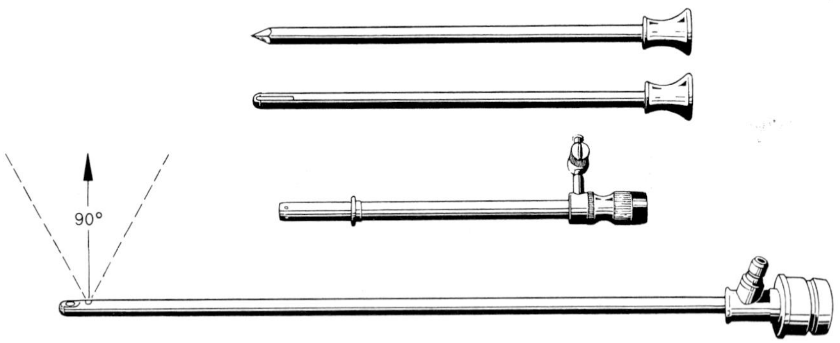


*Figure 12–2.* Culdoscopic instruments. From top down: sharp trochar, dull trochar, cannula, and Wolf fiber optic culdoscope.

the balloon is inflated with sterile water (3 ml.). A self-retaining tubal patency cannula may be substituted for the Foley catheter.

(e) Creation of a minimal pneumoperitoneum prior to the introduction of the trochar: An 18-gauge spinal needle attached to a 10-cc. syringe with the barrel removed or a small Clyman trochar (Fig. 12–1, *F*) is inserted through the cul-de-sac. When a free cul-de-sac is identified, air will be heard rushing in.

(f) The trochar is fitted into the cannula and thrust through the vagina between the uterosacral ligaments into the cul-de-sac.

(g) When the trochar is removed, air again will be heard rushing into the peritoneal cavity.

(h) At this point, the Sims speculum is removed.

(i) The culdoscope is introduced through the cannula, and the fiber optic bundle or light cord is attached (Fig. 12–3).

(j) Following completion of the examination, the culdoscope and tenaculum are removed. The Foley catheter or patency cannula is removed. At this time it is

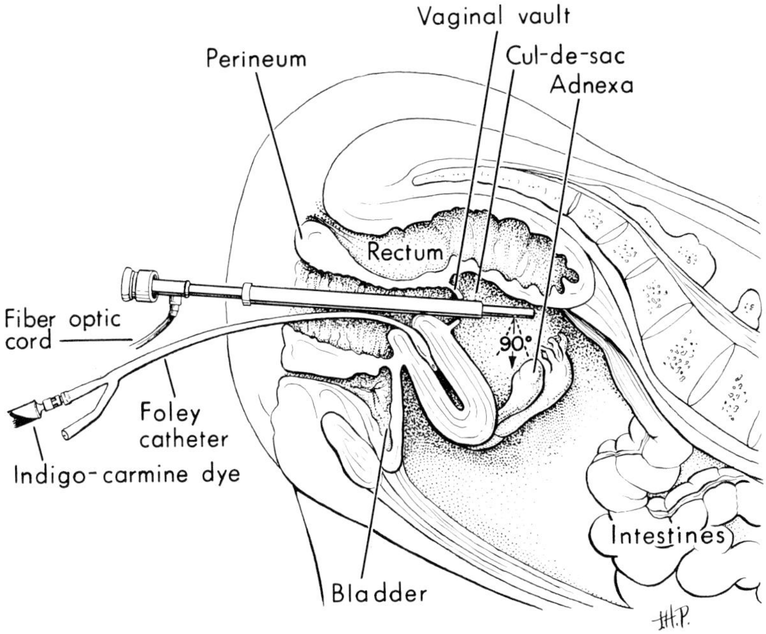


*Figure 12–3.* Modus operandi of culdoscopy. Cross section of patient in knee-chest position with culdoscope in place in the cul-de-sac and Foley catheter in utero.

*The Fertility Institute*

CULDOSCOPY

Name__________Pt. No.__________Date__________
Surgeon__________Assistant__________Adm. No.__________
Pre-op Diag. LMP__________Cycle Day____

L.

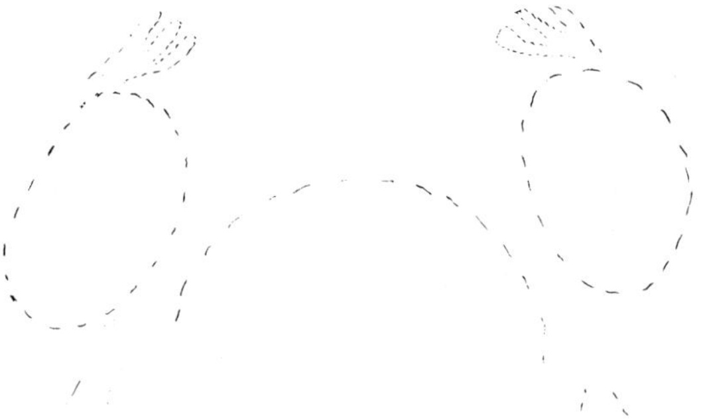

R.

PERITONEUM:
UTERUS: Size Shape Color
Abnormalities
Pathology
Uterosacral Lig.

R. OVARY: Size Shape Color Blood Vessels
Surface: Smooth Tunic Follicles
Wrinkled
Luteal Tissue
Abnormalities
Utero-Ovarian Ligament

L. OVARY: Size Shape Color Blood Vessels
Surface: Smooth Tunic Follicles
Wrinkled
Luteal Tissue
Abnormalities
Utero-Ovarian Ligament

R. TUBE: Length Color Surface
Fimbria Patency Movement Peristalsis

L. TUBE: Length Color Surface
Fimbria Patency Movement Peristalsis

PHOTOGRAPHS: Voltage Exposure Film #

MORBIDITY:

THERAPY:
Response:

PATHOLOGY:

*Figure 12–4.* Culdoscopy form, on which observations are quickly and accurately recorded for future reference.

possible to perform endometrial biopsy or curettage in the knee-chest position. These procedures may be delayed until the patient is in lithotomy position.

(k) The surgeon's hand compresses the abdomen, and the patient is placed in prone position. In this manner most of the air can be expressed from the abdominal cavity. The cannula is then removed. It is usually unnecessary to suture the vaginal vault unless bleeding occurs.

5. Recording and illustrations of observations.
   The form illustrated in Figure 12–4 is filled out. Data obtained and recorded in this way are quite useful.
6. Postculdoscopy orders.
   (a) The patient may be ambulated as soon as the effects of the sedation subside.
   (b) Coitus and douches are prohibited for one week.
   (c) Prophylactic antibiotic therapy is rarely given.

The view obtained at culdoscopy differs from that seen at laparoscopy. (See Chapter 17.) A panoramic view of the internal genitalia may or may not be obtainable, and it is usually necessary to rotate the culdoscope both clockwise and counterclockwise to visualize pelvic structures.

Decker stated that the fallopian tubes, ovaries, anterior and posterior walls of the uterus, sigmoid, rectum, broad ligament, sacral ligament, promontory of the sacrum, the small bowel, and sometimes the appendix may be seen. However, these are not always visualized in each case. Frequently, the anterior uterine wall, the cul-de-sac, and uterosacral ligaments are not clearly seen. Typically, only the fimbriae of the fallopian tubes are clearly discernible. A clear picture of the ovaries is usually obtained. It is possible to establish tubal patency by injecting a dilute solution of indigo carmine or methylene blue dyes through the previously placed Foley catheter or cannula.

### *Culdoscopy and the Obese Patient*

Although the obese patient is difficult to examine bimanually, she is frequently a good candidate for culdoscopy. However, the obese patient is not a particularly good candidate for any type of surgical procedure. I recently subjected a very obese patient with amenorrhea to culdoscopy and was able to visualize ovaries compatible with the Stein-Leventhal syndrome. Having made this diagnosis, I was loathe to prescribe definitive treatment to stimulate ovulation, and the surgical approach of ovarian resection would have been inadvisable. Furthermore, this patient would have been a very poor candidate for a pregnancy. However, at least the diagnosis was made, and if substantial weight reduction were possible, definitive treatment could be instituted.

### *Culdoscopy and Curettage*

It is very simple to combine curettage with culdoscopy. During anesthesia performed for culdoscopy, in addition to infiltrating the cul-de-sac with an anesthetic solution, we routinely infiltrate the uterosacral ligaments and parametrium. This is done so that the cervical canal may be dilated and a patency cannula or a Foley catheter inserted. Also, further dilatation of the cervix and curettage is easily performed. Although it is possible to do a curettage or endometrial biopsy on a patient in the knee-chest position, it is our preference to place the patient in a prone position, evacuating the pneumoperitoneum before proceeding. The patient is placed in lithotomy or gynecologic position, and the curettage proceeds in the usual manner. The nerve block is usually adequate for the entire procedure of curettage, though the occasional sensitive patient may require brief nitrous oxide analgesia in addition.

### *Complications*

There have been few complications following culdoscopy in our series, and these occurred during our initial experience and have diminished in number with progressive improvement in technical skill. We have observed single instances of (1) traumatic rectal bleeding, (2) bleeding due to necrosis of the posterior lip of the cervix from the use of a double-toothed tenaculum, (3) bleeding from the vaginal puncture site, (4) mediastinal emphysema due to the use of a large experimental pelvic endoscope, and (5) perirenal air insufflation due to failure of penetration into the free peritoneal cavity. Local or systemic signs of inflammation rarely occur. Rectal perforation has occurred several times with prompt healing.

Postoperatively, the patient has little discomfort when lying horizontally, but she may experience shoulder pain since it is usually impossible to remove all the air created by the pneumoperitoneum.

Bleeding from the cul-de-sac puncture rarely occurs, but the area should be inspected before the patient is discharged, to make sure that excessive vaginal bleeding does not occur. The bleeding site can be easily visualized and secured with a single catgut stitch.

The patient should be instructed in advance, preferably in the doctor's office, concerning position she will be required to assume on the operating room table. Decker suggests a screening examination in which the patient is placed in knee-chest position on the office examining table. A Sims speculum is used to expose the posterior fornix, and the ballooning sign is demonstrated. This is characterized by the posterior fornix stretching into a taut, smooth, concave drum. When in doubt, it is possible to puncture the cul-de-sac with a needle or thin trochar to determine whether a pneumoperitoneum can be induced with a small amount of air. The sound of air entering the cul-de-sac is usually audible; if there is any doubt, the patient should be allowed to assume the erect posture to determine whether or not shoulder pain occurs as in a Rubin test.

## CULDOSCOPIC PHOTOGRAPHY

Cohen and Guterman, in 1953, described a pelvic photoscope and obtained Kodachrome transparencies, excellent in quality but only 6 mm. in diameter. The photoscope and cannula were 14.5 mm. in diameter, and suture of the perforation site was required after each examination. This incandescent scope was clearly impractical.

In 1963, Clyman described a new Pan Culdoscope-Diagnostic, which had both photographic and operative potentials. This instrument utilized an improved optical system and had an incandescent lamp, the voltage of which could be increased. The overloading of the lamp voltage was necessary to increase illumination at the time of photography. Clyman was able to adapt any single lens reflex camera for still photographs and he used the Camex 8 mm. single lens reflex movie camera for cinematography. He has since changed to a fiber optic system. Clyman also utilized a variety of instruments for biopsy, aspiration of cysts, and cautery. Balin, Wan, and Israel

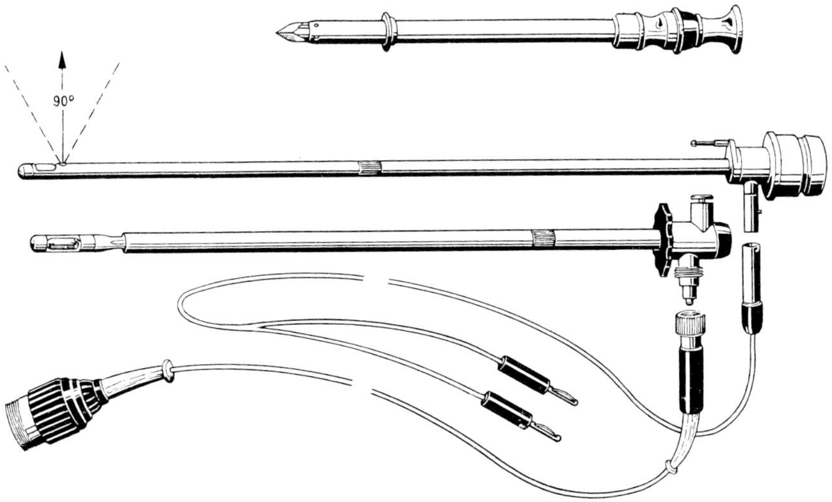


*Figure 12–5.* Wolf flash culdoscope. From top down: trochar and cannula, 8 mm. Wolf incandescent 90° culdoscope, flash lamp carrier sleeve, and flash and light cords.

(1966) documented the various techniques useful for cinematography, still photography and television at culdoscopy.

We have obtained superior photographs with the Richard Wolf culdoscope with electronic flash (Fig. 12–5). Our technique is as follows: Culdoscopy is performed using the Wolf 7 mm. culdoscope with incandescent lamp through an 8 mm. cannula (Fig. 12–1, *H* and *J*). Should photography be desired, the culdoscope and cannula are removed from the cul-de-sac perforation and a larger trochar and cannula introduced. This cannula is of sufficient size to accept a sleeve containing a miniature electronic flash bulb. The culdoscope is inserted through this sleeve and locked in place, and the cord for the incandescent light and the large insulated cord for the electronic flash are attached. The single lens reflex camera is attached to the culdoscope and a still photograph obtained.

Excellent photographs, measuring 17 mm. in diameter, have been obtained with Ektachrome X daylight film, ASA rating 64, in a Leicaflex camera having a lens with a focal length of 110 mm. Transparencies measuring 9 mm. may be obtained with the Pen F camera and a 75 mm. lens. This camera exposes one-half of each frame of the 35 mm. film at a time. Still photographs may also be obtained with high speed Ektachrome at one-fifteenth or one-thirtieth of a second exposure.

Sixteen millimeter movies may be obtained at culdoscopy with the Wolf fiber optic culdoscope or the Decker photographic culdoscope with a 1000 watt fiber optic power supply. We use the Beaulieu camera with a 25 mm. lens plus Ektachrome daylight film, ASA rating 160.

*Chapter Thirteen*

# CULDOSCOPY VERSUS LAPAROSCOPY

## PRESENTATION

Culdoscopy, or transvaginal pelvic endoscopy, is an American invention and is favored by American gynecologists. Laparoscopy (peritoneoscopy, celioscopy), the method of endoscopic visualization of the peritoneal cavity through the anterior abdominal wall, predates culdoscopy and, being a European invention, is favored by European gynecologists. In a previous publication (Cohen, 1968*a*) I compared the two techniques (Fig. 13–1) and reported my experiences with 102 laparoscopies.

It is appropriate now to compare 300 cases each of culdoscopy and laparoscopy as to indications, contraindications, complications, patient acceptance, and ease of visualization. This series of culdoscopies and laparoscopies constitutes my personal experience at Michael Reese Hospital during the past several years. I shall henceforth use the term gynecologic endoscopy to include both culdoscopy and laparoscopy.

The patients' ages in the two series varied from 12 to 85 years (Table 13–1). The range in the culdoscopy series was 18 to 55 years; in the laparoscopy series, 12 to 85 years. Table 13–2 lists the indications for culdoscopy and laparoscopy, respectively. Primary or secondary infertility was the chief indication in both series.

Table 13–3 presents the gynecologic endoscopic findings in primary and secondary infertile patients obtained with the two techniques. Among the 243 infertile patients subjected to culdoscopy, pelvic inflammatory disease and endometriosis were seen most fre-

| | CULDOSCOPY | LAPAROSCOPY |
|---|---|---|
| PATIENT POSITION | KNEE-CHEST | LITHOTOMY |
| USUAL ANESTHESIA | LOCAL | GENERAL OR INNOVAR* & LOCAL |
| PNEUMOPERITONEUM | SPONTANEOUS (AIR) | INDUCED 1 - 4 LITERS $CO_2$, $O_2$, or $N_2O$ |

VIEW

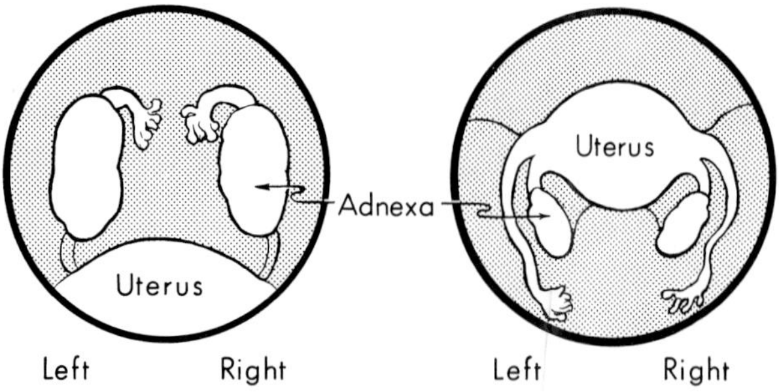


*McNeil Laboratories, Inc., Fort Washington, Pa.

*Figure 13–1.* Culdoscopic view (*left*) compared with panorama obtained at gynecologic laparoscopy (*right*). (Modified from Cohen, M. R. [1968*a*]: Culdoscopy vs. peritoneoscopy. Obstet. Gynec. *31*:310.)

quently; 80 patients were entirely normal. Fifty patients demonstrated ovulation failure. A total of 259 infertile patients were examined by laparoscopy. In these the residue of pelvic inflammatory disease and endometriosis were most frequently found; 69 patients were entirely normal. Ovulation failure occurred in 42 patients.

Table 13–4 shows gynecologic endoscopic findings in both series among patients with pelvic pain.

Table 13–5 shows the gynecologic endoscopic findings in cases of suspected ectopic pregnancy. Culdoscopy was used in 21 patients with a diagnosis of suspected unruptured ectopic pregnancy. In 12 of

**Table 13–1.** Age Distribution for Gynecologic Endoscopy

| AGES | CULDOSCOPY | LAPAROSCOPY |
|---|---|---|
| 20 or Less | 3 | 11 |
| 21–30 | 208 | 208 |
| 31–40 | 79 | 63 |
| 41–50 | 9 | 11 |
| Over 50 | 1 | 7 |
| Total | 300 | 300 |

**Table 13–2.** Indications for Gynecologic Endoscopy

| | CULDOSCOPY (300 Patients) | LAPAROSCOPY (300 Patients) |
|---|---|---|
| Primary infertility | 180 | 177 |
| Secondary infertility | 63 | 82 |
| Pelvic pain | 7 | 14 |
| Suspected ectopic pregnancy | 21 | 9 |
| Metrorrhagia | 16 | 2 |
| Amenorrhea (exclusive of infertile patients) | 13 | 2 |
| Pelvic mass | – | 7 |
| Vaginal atresia | – | 1 |
| Suspected carcinoma of tube | – | 1 |
| Tubal sterilization | – | 5 |

these a tubal pregnancy was disclosed. In six such patients, laparoscopy uncovered one tubal pregnancy.

Table 13–6 lists technical difficulties encountered in these series of gynecologic endoscopies. It was impossible to subject five of the patients to culdoscopy. We experienced only one laparoscopy failure in all 300 patients. However, there was incomplete pelvic visualization of 30 patients by culdoscopy and of 37 patients by laparoscopy. With culdoscopy we expect to visualize at most the distal half of each

**Table 13–3.** Gynecologic Endoscopic Findings in Infertile Patients

| | CULDOSCOPY | | LAPAROSCOPY | |
|---|---|---|---|---|
| | *Primary Infertility (180 Patients)* | *Secondary Infertility (63 Patients)* | *Primary Infertility (177 Patients)* | *Secondary Infertility (82 Patients)* |
| Negative findings | 57 | 23 | 44 | 25 |
| Adhesions (Pelvic inflammatory disease) | 59 | 23 | 52 | 25 |
| Endometriosis | 30 | 13 | 46 | 14 |
| Fibroids | 22 | 5 | 20 | 6 |
| Tubal occlusion | 16 | 10 | 22 | 8 |
| Tubal phimosis | 1 | – | 1 | 3 |
| Stein-Leventhal syndrome | 15 | 3 | 14 | 8 |
| Resting ovaries | 3 | – | 2 | – |
| Wrinkled ovaries | – | 1 | 2 | 1 |
| Simple cyst of ovary | 9 | – | 5 | 1 |
| Corpus luteum cyst | 3 | – | 2 | 2 |
| Double uterus | 1 | – | – | 1 |
| Sclerotic ovaries | – | – | 1 | – |
| Acute anteflexion of uterus | 3 | – | – | – |
| Hypoplastic uterus | 1 | – | – | – |
| Ovulation failure | 40 | 10 | 36 | 6 |

**Table 13–4.** Gynecologic Endoscopic Findings in Patients with Pelvic Pain

| | CULDOSCOPY *(7 Patients)* | LAPAROSCOPY *(14 Patients)* |
|---|---|---|
| Endometriosis | 2 | 5 |
| Chronic pelvic inflammatory disease | 2 | 6 |
| Fibroids | 2 | 3 |
| Normal | 2 | 6 |
| Simple cyst | 1 | 1 |
| Technically impossible | 1 | – |

**Table 13–5.** Gynecologic Endoscopic Findings in Suspected Ectopic Pregnancy

| | CULDOSCOPY *(21 Patients)* | LAPAROSCOPY *(6 Patients)* |
|---|---|---|
| Negative | 3 | 3 |
| Other pathologic conditions | 6 | 2 |
| Tubal pregnancy | 12 | 1 |

**Table 13–6.** Technical Difficulties in Gynecologic Endoscopy

| | CULDOSCOPY | LAPAROSCOPY |
|---|---|---|
| Failure of technique | 5 | 1 |
| Incomplete pelvic visualization | 30 | 37 |
| Laparoscopies performed when culdoscopy was contraindicated | – | 66 |
| Culdoscopies performed when laparoscopy was contraindicated | 1 | – |

**Table 13–7.** Complications During Gynecologic Endoscopy

| | CULDOSCOPY | LAPAROSCOPY |
|---|---|---|
| Anesthesia | 1 | 2 |
| Subperitoneal gas | – | 7 |
| Bleeding | 1 | 3 |
| Acute pelvic inflammatory disease | 1 | – |
| Omental emphysema | – | 1 |

fallopian tube, both ovaries, and the posterior aspect of the uterus. Visualization of uterosacral ligaments is difficult. The laparoscopist, on the other hand, expects to visualize the fallopian tubes completely, both ovaries, the uterosacral ligaments and cul-de-sac, and all surfaces of the uterus. There were 66 laparoscopies in patients in whom culdoscopy was contraindicated, chiefly because of obliteration of the cul-de-sac, fixed retroversion, or cul-de-sac mass. In addition, one child had a rudimentary vagina, and an 85-year-old patient had atrophic external genitalia. The pelvic mass, palpated bimanually, was retroperitoneal and could not be visualized. One culdoscopy was performed in a situation where laparoscopy was contraindicated because of extensive abdominal scars.

Table 13–7 lists complications encountered in both techniques. Extreme nausea and vomiting occurred in one patient after culdoscopy, and this was attributed to drug sensitivity. Two complications due to anesthesia occurred in our group of laparoscopies. In one, spinal anesthesia was used because of the presence of severe pulmonary emphysema. Severe hypotension resulted, and the anesthesiologist refused to put the patient in a sufficiently steep Trendelenburg position for adequate visualization. The second patient developed tachycardia and gallop rhythm due to overdistention of the abdomen with carbon dioxide gas. When the gas was allowed to escape, the pulse came back to normal. Carbon dioxide was injected subperitoneally in seven patients. This subperitoneal gas had to be evacuated before a proper pneumoperitoneum could be estab-

**Table 13–8.** Methods of Anesthesia

| | CULDOSCOPY | LAPAROSCOPY |
|---|---|---|
| Local | 299 | 1 |
| Pudendal block | 1 | – |
| Spinal | – | 5 |
| General | – | 264 |
| Innovar plus local | – | 21 |
| Innovar plus $N_2O$ | – | 9 |

**Table 13–9.** Adjuvant Procedures During Laparoscopy

| | NUMBER OF PATIENTS |
|---|---|
| Ovarian biopsy | 7 |
| Cautery of endometriosis | 3 |
| Lysis of adhesion | 14 |
| Tubal sterilization | 5 |

lished. In one extremely obese patient establishment of pneumoperitoneum transtubally was deemed necessary. Bleeding occurred in three patients during the course of laparoscopy. In one patient there was trauma to a corpus hemorrhagicum; in the other two, bleeding occurred from a perforation of an abdominal wall blood vessel. In each case laparotomy was performed and the bleeding site secured. One patient developed an acute pelvic inflammatory disease after culdoscopy that was controlled with antibiotics. Late bleeding from the culdoscopy wound necessitated suturing in one patient.

Table 13–8 lists the types of anesthesia for both procedures. Local anesthesia was the procedure of choice in culdoscopy, while general anesthesia was preferred in laparoscopy. Patient acceptance for both procedures has been excellent.

Adjuvant procedures performed during laparoscopy are listed in Table 13–9. These were discussed in Chapter 11.

I have previously described still photography with electronic flash and cinematography during laparoscopy. Inasmuch as the endoscope is inserted through the abdominal wall some distance from the pelvic organs, panoramic views may be easily obtained. During culdoscopy a panoramic view is more difficult to obtain because the scope is very close to the organs being viewed. Both still photography and cinematography may be performed utilizing fiber optics with a powerful 1000 watt power supply.*

## DISCUSSION

For the gynecologist interested in the diagnosis of the infertile female, we urge that the techniques of culdoscopy or laparoscopy be employed. Both techniques have a great deal to offer in the diagnosis of obscure pelvic conditions. One advantage of culdoscopy is that it is a less traumatic procedure, inasmuch as local anesthesia may be

*Eder Instrument Company, Chicago, Ill.

employed. Laparoscopy frequently requires a brief, although deep, surgical anesthesia. Although laparoscopy may be performed under local anesthesia plus neuroleptanalgesia, an experienced anesthetist is required (Chapter 4). The view obtained at culdoscopy is more limited in scope. Usually only the tips of the fallopian tubes, the surfaces of the ovary and the posterior wall of the uterus are visualized. The view obtained at laparoscopy is more easily learned by the novice since this view resembles that seen at laparotomy. All surfaces of the uterus, the cul-de-sac, uterosacral ligaments, and the entire length of the fallopian tubes and ovaries may be visualized. It is frequently necessary to insert a probe through the abdominal wall so that the adnexal structures may be brought into view.

One patient with extensive abdominal wall scarring from prior surgery underwent culdoscopy with ease, whereas laparoscopy would have been impossible. Of the 300 laparoscopies, 66 were performed in patients in whom culdoscopy was contraindicated. Advocates of culdoscopy have stated that should there be a contraindication to this technique, such as a fixed retroversion or cul-de-sac mass, laparotomy would be mandatory; hence, they do not recognize a need for laparoscopy. However, such pelvic findings could be due to endometriosis for which medical treatment might be more beneficial. Laparoscopy is preferred whenever endometriosis is suspected, even with a free cul-de-sac, because the true nature and extent of the disease can be better visualized. We prefer the technique of laparoscopy in the presence of amenorrhea so that ovarian biopsies may be obtained.

We have recently begun to perform tubal sterilization by means of the Steptoe technique (Chapter 10). Thus far it has been a simple and rewarding procedure. We intend to utilize this method further for permanent interval tubal sterilization via laparoscopy.

At Michael Reese Hospital we are training residents in both techniques. We have found it easier to teach the technique of laparoscopy than culdoscopy, and certainly pelvic anatomy is easier to demonstrate at laparoscopy. Our present resident group prefers laparoscopy to culdoscopy. In comparing visualization of the pelvic organs via gynecologic endoscopy, there were 30 patients in whom culdoscopy was not completely satisfactory, as opposed to 37 similar cases in the laparoscopy group. The majority of these 37 cases occurred during our early experience with laparoscopy and were unsatisfactory because of improper pneumoperitoneum, loss of gas, and improper positioning of the patient on the table.

Complications with either technique were few. With laparoscopy we had seven patients in whom there was difficulty in creating the pneumoperitoneum. The subperitoneal gas was evacuated and a proper pneumoperitoneum performed in each of these cases. Most complications reported in the literature have occurred while creating the pneumoperitoneum prior to laparoscopy.

## CONCLUSIONS

1. The indications for culdoscopy and for laparoscopy are the same, and either technique may be utilized for the diagnosis of obscure pelvic diseases.
2. Laparoscopy is especially useful when culdoscopy is contraindicated. In our series of 300 cases, 66 laparoscopies were performed in cases in which culdoscopies would have been contraindicated.
3. Complications were minimal in both techniques.
4. With laparoscopy the following surgical procedures were employed:
   (a) Lysis of fine pelvic adhesions.
   (b) Cautery of endometrial implant.
   (c) Tubal sterilization.
   (d) Ovarian biopsy.
5. Photography in color may be routinely performed for proper documentation of findings in both culdoscopy and laparoscopy.

*Chapter Fourteen*

# ENDOSCOPY AND THE INFERTILE FEMALE

Gynecologic endoscopy is indicated in every infertile patient 30 years of age or older and in any patient, regardless of age, infertile for three years or more. This enthusiastic endorsement is based on a wide experience which has provided me with evidence proving the value of endoscopy under these circumstances.

In order to interpret observations during laparoscopy or culdoscopy one must first be familiar with the normal gross anatomy of the pelvic structures. Secondly, one must be able to recognize the appearance of the pelvic organs of reproduction during the various phases of the menstrual cycle.

The optimal time for performing laparoscopy or culdoscopy in the infertile female is immediately after ovulation has occurred. With failure of ovulation, on the other hand, it may be done at any time during a period of amenorrhea. Although numerous tests of ovulation have been suggested, e.g., the Farris rat test, glucose reaction, and vaginal smear cytology, at the Fertility Institute we rely chiefly on the basal body temperature chart and cervical mucorrhea (Fig. 14–1).

The woman is instructed to take her basal body temperature, rectally if possible, each morning before rising, beginning shortly after a menstrual period is over and continuing daily until menstruation ensues. She is instructed to report to the office daily from the ninth to the fifteenth day of a typical 28-day cycle. A patient with an irregular cycle may have to be seen more frequently over a longer period. A vaginal speculum is inserted without lubrication and the following routine is performed: the tip of a glass or metal cannula is inserted into the endocervix and, by means of gentle suction, a quantity of endocervical mucus is obtained for examination. This is

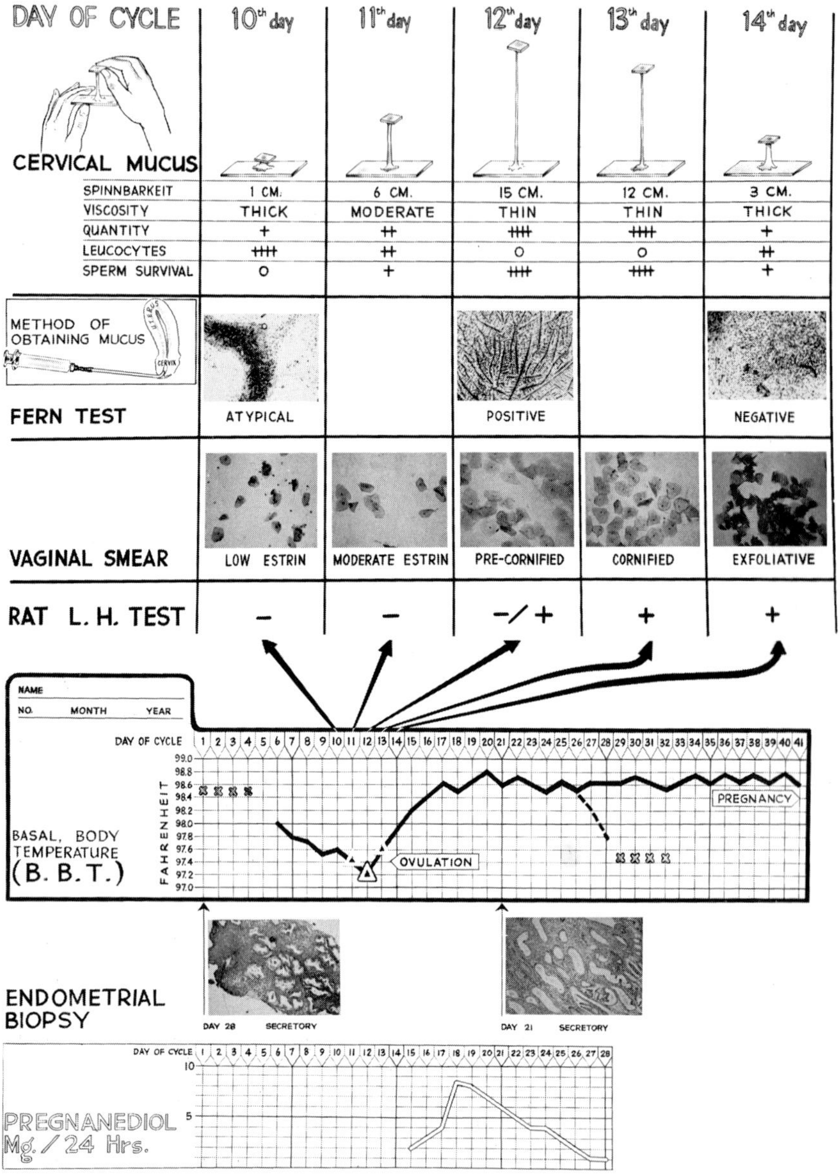


*Figure 14–1.* Clinical criteria of presumptive ovulation, including examination of cervical mucus, vaginal smear, basal body temperature, endometrial biopsy and pregnanediol, related to date of menstrual cycle. (From Cohen, M. R. [1958]: Sterility and infertility: medical views. J.A.M.A. *168*:15.)

blown out on a glass slide, and the amount is estimated from 0 to 4+ (profuse). A glass cover slip is placed on this glob of mucus and the *Spinnbarkeit*, or stretch phenomenon, is measured in centimeters. The cover slip is replaced and the slide examined for the presence of white blood cells and spermatozoa. The cover slip is again removed, the mucus is allowed to dry, and the fern-leaf reaction, or crystallization of the cervical mucus, is noted.

We believe that ovulation occurs at the low point in the temperature cycle, on the day before this low point, or on the rise from low to high. Prior to ovulation the cervical mucus becomes profuse and thin and shows a stretch phenomenon from 10 to 20 cm. in length. Normally at this time large numbers of spermatozoa are recovered postcoitally.

After ovulation occurs, the body temperature becomes elevated and sustained, and the cervical mucus becomes scantier in quantity, thickens, and shows very little Spinnbarkeit. Results of crystallization or the fern test are usually positive during the mucorrhea phase of the cycle.

By utilizing the indirect criteria of ovulation (basal body temperature, vaginal smear, cervical mucus changes, sperm survival), we have found it possible to time the endoscopic examination so that the ovary can be observed in either the preovulative or postovulative state. In the preovulative state, the mature follicle appears as a domed vesicle, bluish in color and approximately 1 cm. in diameter. It is sharply demarcated from the rest of the ovary and occasionally there are small blood vessels coursing over the surface of the bleb.

If ovulation occurs, this structure is replaced by a corpus hemorrhagicum within 24 hours. The corpus hemorrhagicum appears to be larger than the parent follicle, occupying from one-fourth to one-half of the entire ovary and measuring 1.5 to 3 cm. in diameter. The corpus hemorrhagicum is intensely red, is not sharply demarcated from the rest of the ovary, and may have a stigma or clotted blood on its surface. On some occasions the interior of the corpus hemorrhagicum has a dark purplish homogeneous appearance. Later in the cycle this structure takes on a yellowish-red appearance and is more sharply demarcated from the rest of the ovary. The appearance of the mature corpus luteum is well known, but it must be differentiated from a luteinized follicle, which is sharply demarcated and frequently irregular in outline; it rarely exceeds 1 cm. in diameter and has a characteristic pale yellow appearance. Repeated daily culdoscopic observations have enabled us to observe the development of the mature follicle into either a corpus hemorrhagicum or a luteinized follicle. We have observed spontaneous ovulation during the course of culdoscopy and have been able to confirm Decker's (1949) description of the process. The importance of differentiating between the corpus luteum and the luteinized follicle is obvious. Both of these structures may produce similar endometrial patterns, pregnanediol excretion, basal body temperature curves, vaginal smears, and cervical mucus changes. For diagnostic purposes, the direct examination of the ovary through the endoscope is the only practical means of distinguishing these two structures in repeated cycles.

Laparoscopy or culdoscopy is usually scheduled immediately following the mucorrhea phase of the cycle. Figure 14–2 indicates a monthly ovulation record in relation to the optimal time for laparoscopy or culdoscopy. In a patient with a typical 28-day cycle this endoscopic procedure should be performed from day 14 through day 21 of the cycle. Inasmuch as the patient is hospitalized for this endoscopic procedure, it is feasible to obtain an endometrial biopsy, a 24-hour urine collection for pregnanediol and 17-ketosteroids, and

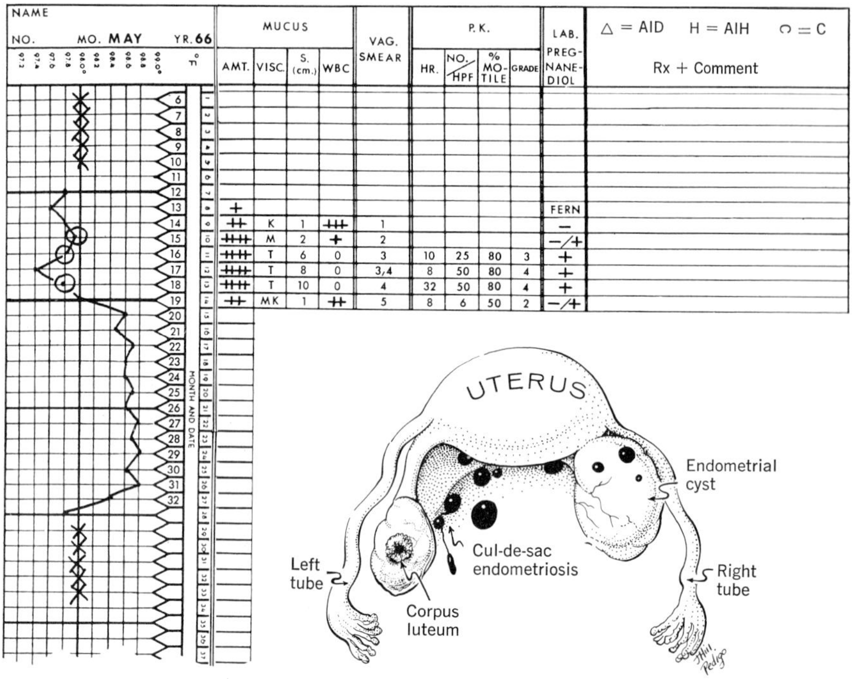


*Figure 14–2.* Ovulation timing followed by culdoscopy or laparoscopy. On basal body temperature chart (*left*), the circle on days 10, 11, and 13 indicates coitus. Under "MUCUS," amount is given as + to ++++. Viscosity ("VISC.") is designated *K*, thick; *M*, moderate; and *T*, thin. *S* indicates Spinnbarkeit in centimeters. *WBC* refers to leukocytes present. Vaginal smear shows degree of estrogenic activity in terms of maturation index (1–4), regression (5–6), or unsuitable for hormone cytology (7). "P.K." indicates postcoital examination of mucus (Sims-Huhner test). Under "LAB.," ferning is indicated as positive (+), negative (−), or atypical (−/+). (From Cohen, M. R. [1968*a*]: Culdoscopy vs. peritoneoscopy. Obstet. Gynec. *31*:310.)

thyroid function tests as routine procedures in the infertile patient. During periods of amenorrhea there is no definite time for performing this technique. However, occasionally the amenorrheic patient may suddenly demonstrate a spurt of mucus with an elevation of the basal body temperature, and in such patients we have been able to obtain visual (endoscopic) evidence of ovulation.

It is essential to test for tubal patency during endoscopy. For this purpose a self-retaining cannula or Foley catheter is inserted through the cervix. Up to 10 cc. of indigo carmine solution (1:5) or methylene blue (1% in saline) are injected. Initially the dye distends the tubes and then escapes drop by drop from the fimbria. When tubes are not patent, one may locate and observe the site of obstruction.

In some patients whose tubal patency has been previously established with insufflation of carbon dioxide, the dye oozes into periovarian and peritubal adhesions before it finds its way into the free peritoneal cavity. Although such tubes may be patent to gas, they may not permit the normal flow of liquids. This demonstrates interference with ovum transfer.

In many infertile patients, periovarian adhesions of varying size, density, and vascularity are seen extending from the sites of follicle rupture to adjacent structures. These adhesions may or may not be associated with early endometriosis, and minimal adhesions apparently are no barrier to fertility. However, a few patients will demonstrate extensive periovarian adhesions which can completely prevent ovum transfer. We know of no other way of evaluating pelvic adhesions than by endoscopy.

Laparoscopy and culdoscopy have been of assistance in distinguishing the appearance of the ovary in various types of menstrual dysfunction. Although the surface characteristics do not necessarily provide an etiological diagnosis, such information does assist the physician in his plan of therapy. In the amenorrheic patient the ovaries may exhibit many variants ranging from complete absence of functional ovarian tissue to the early corpus luteum of pregnancy.

Although the syndrome of gonadal dysgenesis (Turner, 1938) has been described in detail, its diagnosis in the adult may be obscured by previous hormone administration accompanied by the development of secondary sex characteristics. The untreated patient may exhibit the characteristic shortness of stature, lack of secondary sex characteristics, and primary amenorrhea. Endoscopy in these cases reveals a tiny plaque of undifferentiated tissue in the region of each broad ligament. The uterus is tiny and the tubes are long and thin.

Some patients with amenorrhea of long duration have normal secondary sex characteristics, but bimanual examination shows that the uterus is hypoplastic. The endometrium and vaginal smear show absence of estrogenic activity. Endoscopy demonstrates the presence of ovaries that are smaller than normal, smooth-surfaced, white, and have few or no vascular markings and no evidence of follicular activity. The tubes appear normal.

We have observed another group of patients who had secondary amenorrhea of relatively short duration and normal secondary sex characteristics. Bimanual examination reveals normal corpus uteri and at times unilateral ovarian enlargement. The vaginal smear and endometrial pattern reveal persistent estrogenic activity. At culdoscopy or laparoscopy the uterus and tubes appear normal. The ovaries may contain one or more clear follicle cysts.

In a patient in whom there is x-ray evidence of tubal obstruction and in whom laparotomy is contemplated, we frequently perform laparoscopy or culdoscopy as a feasibility study prior to definitive surgery. Should endoscopic visualization disclose such an extensive pathologic condition as to make the surgical procedure impossible, unnecessary laparotomy will have been avoided.

Furthermore, with the infertile patient we advise laparoscopy six months following any laparotomy for infertility if pregnancy does not occur during this time. During this second look, minor pelvic adhesions may be lysed, recurrent endometrial nodules may be cauterized, and patency of the tubes verified. Such an examination also has great prognostic value.

*Chapter Fifteen*

# ENDOSCOPY IN THE DIAGNOSIS AND PROGNOSIS OF THE STEIN-LEVENTHAL SYNDROME

In 1935, Stein and Leventhal described the syndrome of amenorrhea associated with bilateral polycystic ovaries. The syndrome of menstrual irregularity, infertility, masculine-type hirsutism, and, frequently, obesity has been well documented through the years (Figs. 15-1 and 15-2). In 1964, Stein summarized his series of 108 patients extending over a period of 34 years. He reported cyclic menses occurring in 95 per cent of the patients after bilateral wedge resection. Among the 83 women complaining of infertility, 71 or 85 per cent became pregnant, with a total of 181 pregnancies. In this series there were five sets of twins, which is about three times the normal rate of multiple births. Stein further stated that after wedge resection, restoration of fertility is permanent.

## DIAGNOSIS OF THE STEIN-LEVENTHAL SYNDROME

Stein et al. (1949) stated that the diagnosis of bilateral polycystic ovaries is greatly enhanced by the use of pneumoroentgenography (gynecography; see Chapter 16). They were able to demonstrate the bilateral ovarian enlargement by this method when palpable

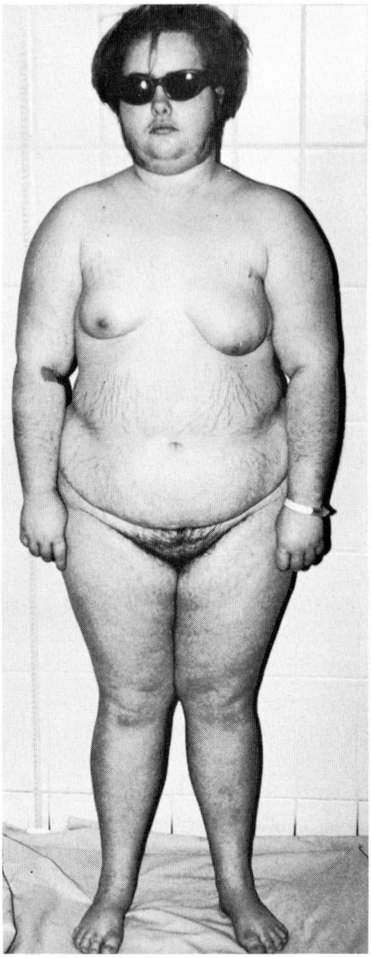

*Figure 15–1.* Patient with secondary amenorrhea, marked hirsutism, obesity, and striae. Laparoscopy demonstrated large bilateral polycystic ovaries. (See Figure 17–18.)

evidence, especially in the obese patient, was in doubt. The shadow of the normal ovary, which is usually about one fourth the size of the uterine corpus, enlarges so that it appears to be from about three fourths to as large as the uterine shadow (Fig. 15–3).

We have found that culdoscopy and laparoscopy are more valuable than gynecography in the diagnosis of the typical bilateral polycystic ovary (Chapter 17). Such an ovary is easily visualized as enlarged, tense, globular or oyster-like in appearance, and having a thickened capsule. A few blood vessels course through this thickened white capsule. Through this capsule one can see what appear to be follicle cysts ranging from 0.5 to 1 cm. in diameter.

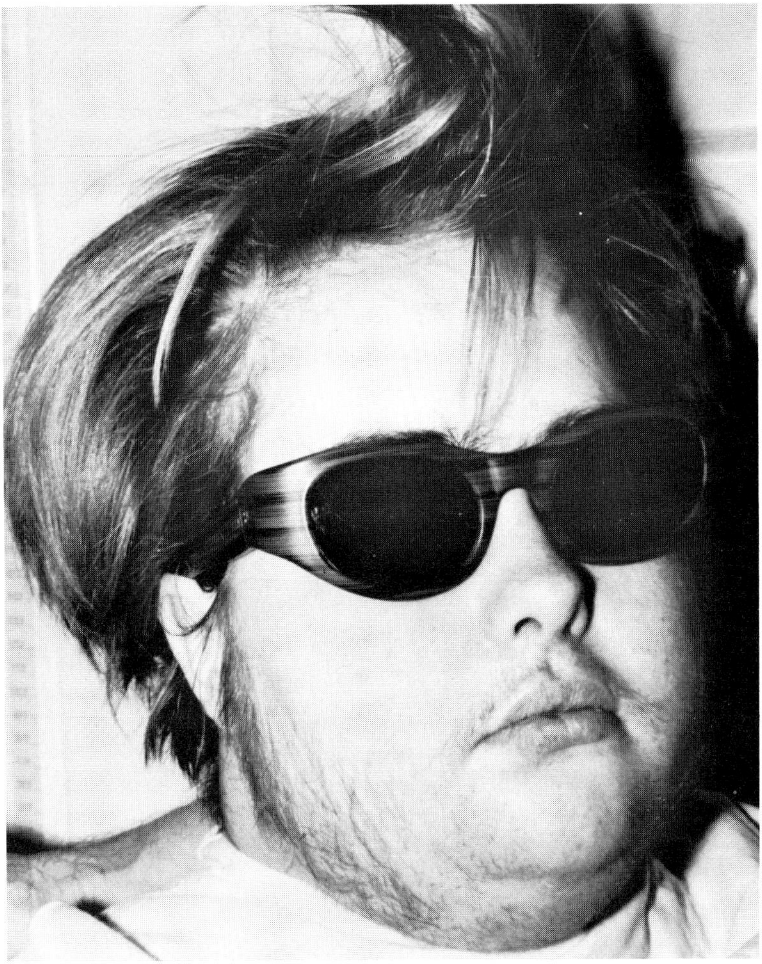

*Figure 15–2.* Photograph of face of same patient in Figure 15–1 showing facial hirsutism.

Frequently small cysts bulge from the surface of the ovary. There is no evidence of recent or old ovulation.

Endometrial biopsy or curettage discloses a proliferative endometrium, especially late proliferative types. Occasionally hyperplastic endometrium may be obtained because of unopposed estrogen secretion. The absence of ovulation may be further documented clinically by a flat basal body temperature curve, a vaginal smear that shows moderate to high estrogenic effect, a moderate amount of mucorrhea with Spinnbarkeit varying from 2 to 4 cm., positive post-coital tests, and positive ferning.

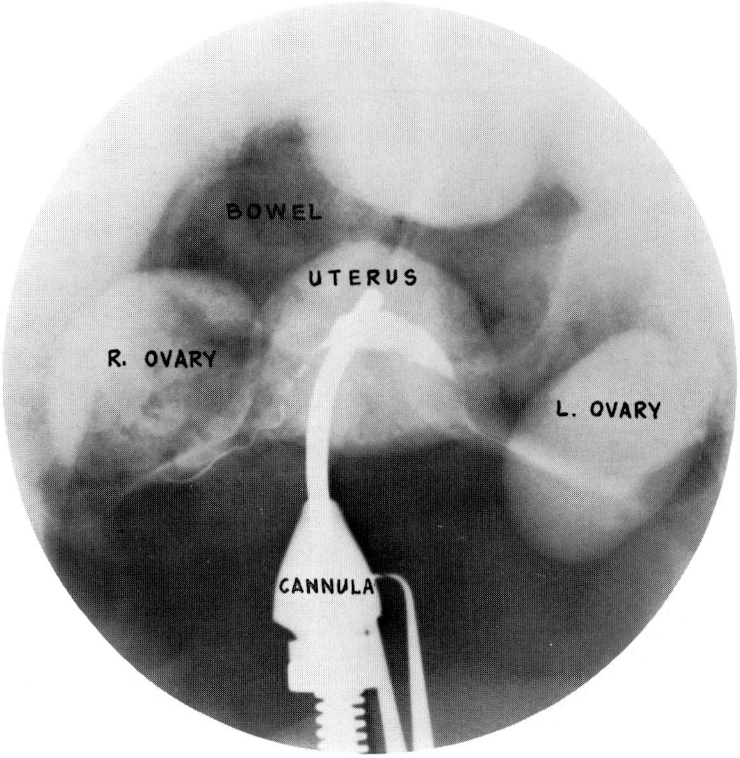


*Figure 15–3.* Bilateral ovarian enlargement typical of Stein-Leventhal syndrome demonstrated by gynecography. (See Chapter 16.)

## TREATMENT OF THE STEIN-LEVENTHAL SYNDROME

Following the report by Greenblatt et al. (1961) concerning use of clomiphene citrate* in the induction of ovulation, it became apparent that this was an effective drug in the treatment of Stein-Leventhal syndrome. In fact, Kistner (1965*a*) advised that it replace the surgical approach as the treatment of choice. Kistner summarized case reports of 1704 patients treated with clomiphene citrate, 391 of whom were considered to have polycystic ovary disease. Of these 391 patients, 305 or 78 per cent responded with evidence of ovulation. Roy and associates (1963), presenting their results on the induction of ovulation with clomiphene citrate in 179 women, reported 35 patients classified as having Stein-Leventhal syndrome. Of these 35 patients, treated during 134 cycles, only 6 had conceptions, although 32 of them ovulated and menstruated during 117 cycles.

*Clomid, Wm. S. Merrell Co., Cincinnati, Ohio

In a comparative study (Cohen, 1966), we reported a group of 29 patients with this syndrome treated with clomiphene citrate during 64 cycles. Forty cycles showed typical diphasic temperature curves. We reported eight pregnancies in seven patients treated with clomiphene. Although our results with clomiphene are not as good as those reported by Stein with ovarian resection, we urge an adequate trial of therapy with this drug before resorting to bilateral ovarian wedge resection. The number of courses of therapy depends largely on whether side effects occur. The occurrence of temporary cystic swelling of the ovaries is not a contraindication to continuation of this therapy, since these cysts disappear in time. In one patient, whose case report is presented in the following section, we chose to resect the ovaries immediately, rather than wait for involution, because of the size of the enlargement and because we were interested in the histopathology of ovarian changes produced by this drug.

Patients with typical polycystic ovaries seem especially sensitive to clomiphene and we urge a trial dose of no more than 50 mg. for five days or less. Prior therapy with clomiphene in no way altered results from bilateral ovarian resection.

Kistner (1965*b*) has suggested that patients who do not respond to clomiphene alone should be treated with injections of human chorionic gonadotropin (HCG). In patients receiving clomiphene therapy there is typically a spurt of mucus which occurs about seven days after the drug therapy is stopped. When this mucorrhea occurs, we perform insemination or urge coitus. The patient is observed the following day for evidence of longevity of spermatozoa. If clomiphene is apparently inducing ovulation and the patient still does not conceive, we give HCG in daily doses varying from 2000 to 10,000 units given intramuscularly at the time of the spurt of mucorrhea and continued daily until thickening of the mucus occurs.

## UNSUCCESSFUL RESULTS FOLLOWING BILATERAL OVARIAN RESECTION AND CLOMIPHENE THERAPY

We have observed patients who have had unsuccessful ovarian resection for Stein-Leventhal syndrome. These patients usually have relatively regular cycles and apparently ovulate, but they remain infertile. Laparoscopy or culdoscopy is useful in evaluating the results of such surgery, and we have found endoscopic evidence of ovarian adhesions extensive enough to prevent ovulation.

Case #12489 is an example of an unsuccessful ovarian resection. Her referring physician wrote:

"Mrs. S. represents a classical example of Stein-Leventhal syndrome. She failed to respond to Clomid [clomiphene] therapy, but conceived on Pergonal, but unfortunately had an obstetric accident which resulted in an intrauterine death. Following this delivery Pergonal became unavailable and the patient was subjected to a bilateral ovarian wedge resection five months ago. Her last visit in October, 1968, revealed that she was now menstruating and ovulating regularly."

The transcript of the hospital record was appended. The surgical pathology report showed wedges of ovarian tissue with thick stroma and cortex, and numerous follicles without evidence of ovulation, consistent with the diagnosis of Stein-Leventhal syndrome.

In a letter dated August 18, 1969, I reported to her referring doctor as follows:

"Inasmuch as Mrs. S. has failed to conceive since her ovarian wedge resection, I hospitalized her for endocrine workup and laparoscopy. My findings, dated July 22, 1969, disclosed extensive adnexal adhe-

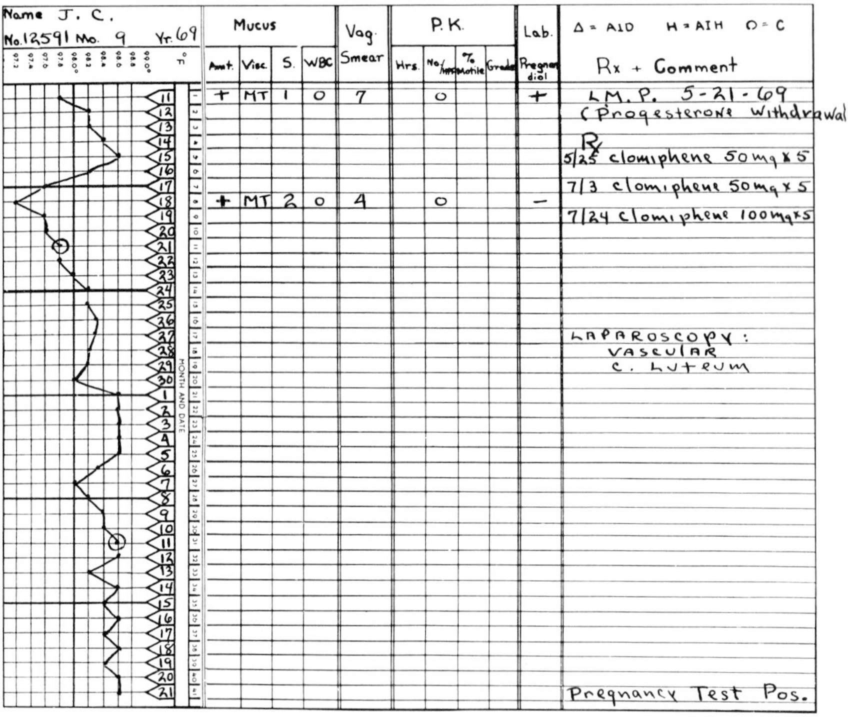


*Figure 15–4.* Ovulation chart of patient J.C. #12591 showing office examinations on 9/11/69 and 9/18/69 and laparoscopy on 9/27/69. Note that three courses of clomiphene had been prescribed; the last course, 100 mg. daily for five days, was begun on 7/24/69. BBT curve was monophasic from 5/21/69 until 9/18/69. (See legend to Figure 14–2.)

*The Fertility Institute*

PERITONEOSCOPY

Name J C. Pt. No. 12591 Date 9-27-69
Surgeon M. R. C. Assistant Adm. No.
Pre-op Diag. LMP 5-21-69 Cycle Day

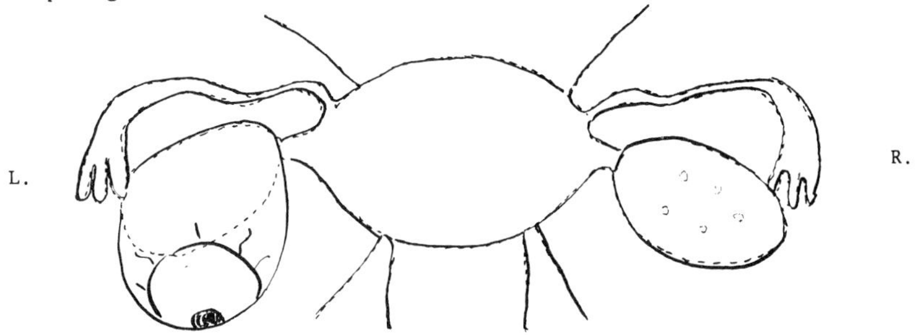


PERITONEUM: Normal (N)
UTERUS: Size N Shape N Color N
Abnormalities O
Pathology O
Uterosacral Lig. N

R. OVARY: Size N Shape N Color white Blood Vessels O
Surface: Smooth ✓ Tunic Thick Follicles Deep
Wrinkled
Luteal Tissue O
Abnormalities O
Utero-Ovarian Ligament N

L. OVARY: Size 4 X N Shape globular Color pink Blood Vessels ✓
Surface: Smooth ✓ Tunic thin Follicles
Wrinkled
Luteal Tissue Mature vascular corp. luteum
Abnormalities O
Utero-Ovarian Ligament N

R. TUBE: Length N Color N Surface N
Fimbria N Patency Movement Peristalsis

L. TUBE: Length N Color N Surface N
Fimbria N Patency Movement Peristalsis

PHOTOGRAPHS: Voltage Exposure Film #
Tech. Difficulty

MORBIDITY:

THERAPY: No biopsy, No patency
Response: Re: possibility of early pregnancy

PATHOLOGY:

*Figure 15–5.* Peritoneoscopy (laparoscopy) sheet, patient J.C. #12591, showing vascular corpus luteum.

sions. Epiploic processes from large bowel partially covered the left ovary and left tube; the right ovary was partially covered with adhesions, as was the fimbria of the right tube. The fimbria of the right tube was definitely phimotic. Although the fimbria of the left tube was not visualized, there was evidence of indigo carmine in the cul-de-sac. I urged that this couple adopt a child, as I could not guarantee that adhesions would not reform after a second laparotomy." (See Figures 17–20 and 17–21.)

Endoscopy has been of value in determining whether a patient really ovulates following resection or after therapy with clomiphene citrate. We have seen evidence of ovulation and of diffuse cystic degeneration and luteinization without ovulation following clomiphene citrate therapy.

Patients with amenorrhea, who are suspected of having the Stein-Leventhal syndrome, report to our office weekly or twice weekly for ovulation timing. We observe such patients very carefully for evidence of changes in cervical mucus correlated with the basal body temperature curve since occasionally spontaneous ovulation without therapy may occur. Should there be clinical evidence of ovulation, endoscopy is useful in confirming the presence of a recent corpus luteum.

We recently observed a patient who had amenorrhea for six months, during which time three courses of clomiphene had been unsuccessful. Our plan was laparoscopy and probable bilateral ovarian wedge resection. At laparoscopy we found evidence of a moderately enlarged ovary on the right with a thickened capsule, typical of the Stein-Leventhal syndrome. The other ovary was globular and enlarged to almost the size of the uterus; the capsule was also thickened. This ovary was rotated with a probe, and to our surprise a very vascular corpus luteum was present on the undersurface. Laparoscopy disclosed that surgical intervention was unnecessary. This ovulation resulted in pregnancy (Figs. 15–4, 15–5, and 17–19).

*Chapter Sixteen*

# GYNECOGRAPHY

Gynecography, a term coined in 1943 by my teacher and former associate, Dr. Irving F. Stein, Sr., refers to a method of silhouetting the female organs by means of a pneumoperitoneum with or without hysterosalpingography. In this procedure carbon dioxide gas is injected through the uterus, as in a Rubin test, or injected by means of a transabdominal needle. After approximately one liter of gas is introduced, the patient is placed in modified knee-chest position and the pelvic organs are visualized utilizing soft tissue x-ray techniques. This simple pneumoperitoneum, when combined with a radiopaque medium, is called complete gynecography. This diagnostic method is useful in delineating ovarian cysts, fibroids, and other intrapelvic pathologic conditions. Experience with pneumoperitoneum is very valuable when one wishes to learn the technique of laparoscopy.

## TECHNIQUE OF GYNECOGRAPHY

Figure 16-1 is an instruction sheet given to patients prior to gynecography. This is a minor surgical procedure performed in the x-ray laboratory and may be used for both inpatient and outpatient cases. Meperidine, 100 mg., is administered intramuscularly or slowly intravenously. The following outlines our routine:

1. The patient is placed in dorsal lithotomy position with her hips elevated on a sand bag.
2. The bladder is catheterized or the patient is instructed to void prior to this examination.
3. A pelvic examination is performed.

X-RAY EXAMINATION OF THE FEMALE ORGANS

The female organs do not photograph when x-rayed unless they are contrasted by gas or a liquid. A simple technique to outline the cavity of the uterus and tubes, and to silhouette the outside of the uterus and ovaries is performed in the x-ray laboratory.

PREPARATION

1. Call for an appointment on the first day of your menstrual period so that the test may be scheduled on day _____ or _____ of your cycle.

2. Take a tap water enema the night before and repeat it the morning of the test.

3. Omit breakfast. (Should the test be scheduled late in the day, eat a light breakfast, but omit lunch.)

4. Have a companion available to escort you home as a sedative is usually administered.

*Figure 16–1.* Instructions to patient for gynecography.

4. A modified Graves speculum is inserted to expose the cervix.
5. The cervix is disinfected.
6. A self-retaining cannula is inserted (Figs. 16–2 and 16–3).
7. The speculum is removed.
8. Pneumoperitoneum is induced transuterinely, as in a Rubin test, or by transabdominal needle. If the Rubin test is positive at 160 mm. of mercury or less, demonstrating patency of at least one fallopian tube, the patient is rotated so that she is in a partial knee-chest position. The table is canted down approximately 15°. One must make sure that the self-retaining cannula has not been disturbed while the patient is rotated to a prone position. The Rubin test is continued until approximately 1000 cc. of carbon dioxide has been instilled.

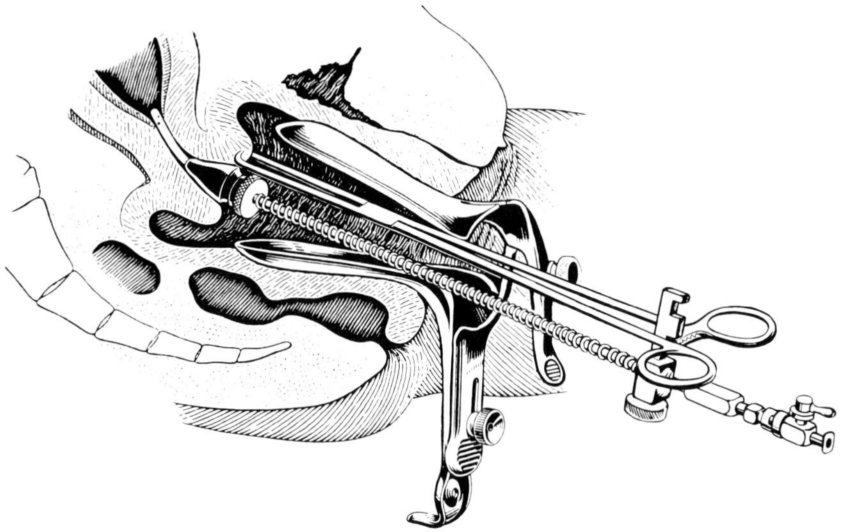

*Figure 16–2.* Modified side-opening Graves speculum exposing cervix. Author's original self-retaining cannula is inserted and fixed with single tenaculum forceps.

The patient's back is arched so that the central ray can be directed between the coccyx and the symphysis pubis and the first x-ray film obtained.

If the tubes are not patent to gas, a pneumoperitoneum is performed transabdominally. (See Chapter 5.) The patient is then rotated and placed in the modified knee-chest position for the first x-ray film. This first pneumoperitoneum film is also a scout film should prior hysterosalpingography have been performed. It is important to inject the carbon dioxide gas rapidly into the peritoneal cavity since this gas is ab-

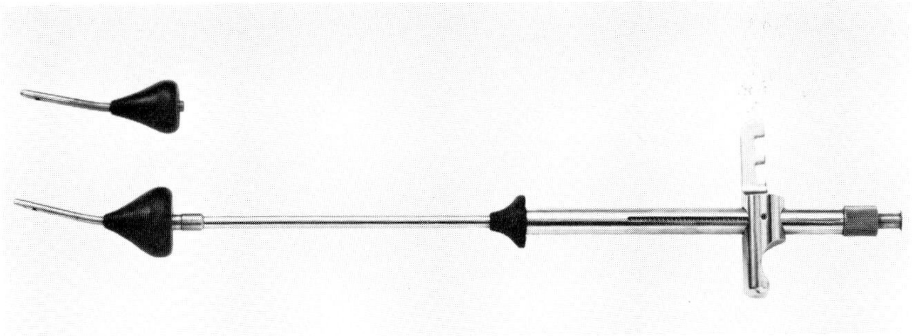

*Figure 16–3.* The author's new self-retaining cannula for hysterosalpingography, tubal insufflation, or gynecography.

**Table 16–1.** X-ray Technique (small focus, 50 ma., 0.8 second, 36 inches distance, Bucky diaphragm)

| Patient's Weight | Body Type | Prone Kvp | Dorsal Kvp |
|---|---|---|---|
| 85 | Gaunt | 56 | 54 |
| 95 | Very thin | 58 | 56 |
| 100 | Thin | 62 | 60 |
| 110 | Thin | 62 | 60 |
| 115 | Thin | 64 | 60 |
| | Average | 66 | 62 |
| 120 | Stocky | 68 | 64 |
| 125 | Average | 66 | 62 |
| 130 | Stocky | 68 | 64 |
| 135 | Stocky | 68 | 64 |
| 140 | Stout | 68 | 64 |
| 150 | Obese | 70 | 66 |
| 185 | Obese | 74 | 72 |
| 205 | Very obese | 76 | 74 |
| 270 | Huge | 86 | 84 |

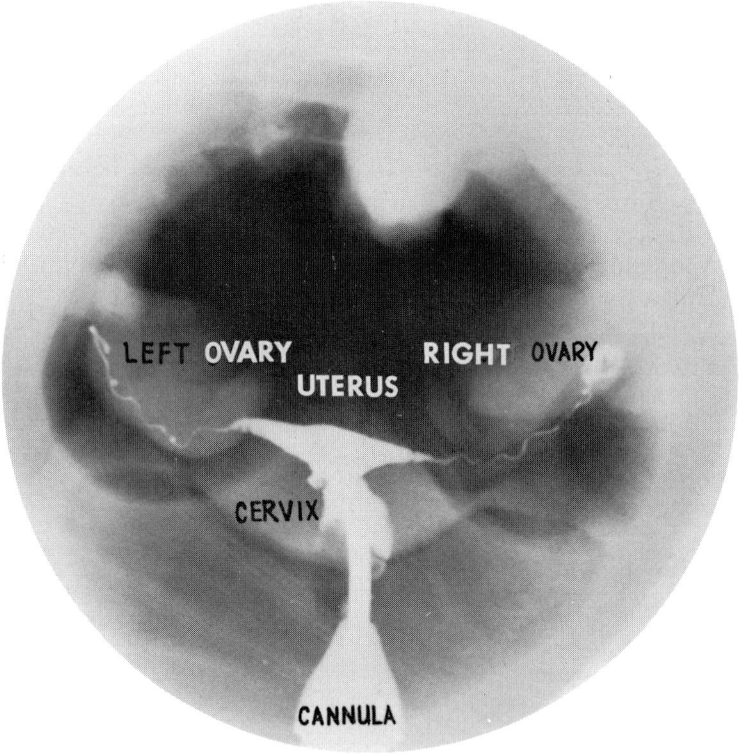


*Figure 16–4.* Complete gynecography, normal genitalia. Pneumoperitoneum outlines pelvic organs; radiopaque dye demonstrates dimensions of uterine cavity and tubal lumina.

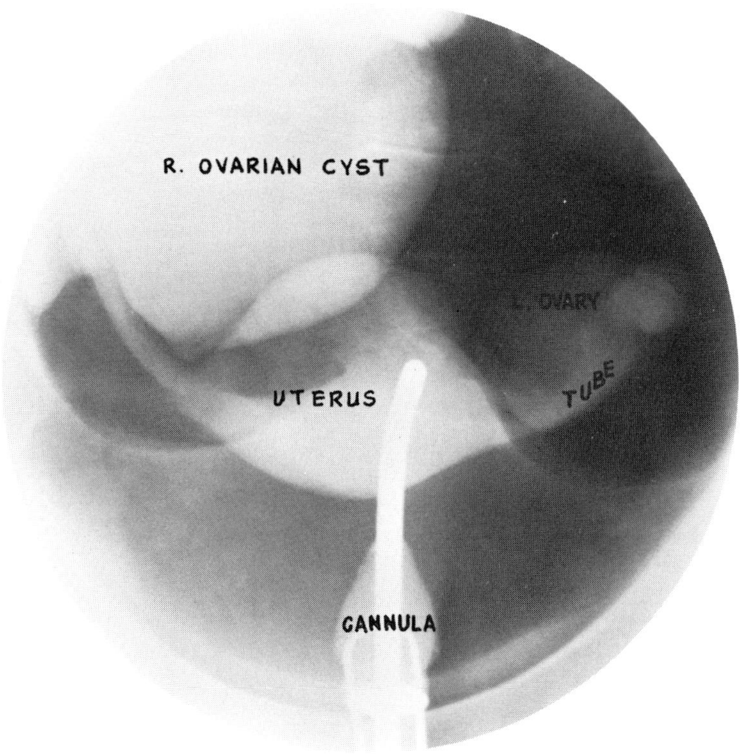


*Figure 16–5.* Transuterine pneumoperitoneum showing large, right ovarian cyst.

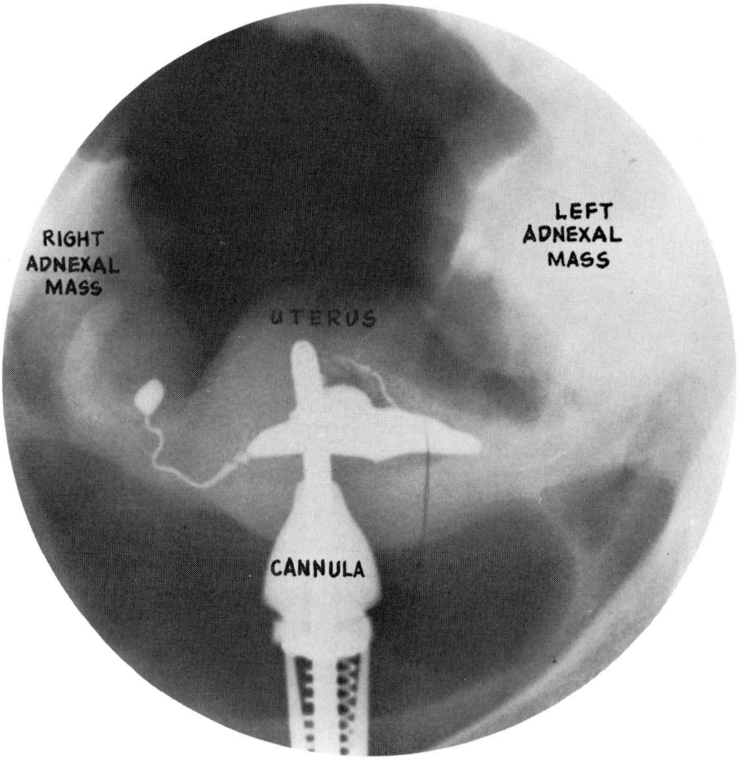


*Figure 16–6.* Complete gynecography in presence of chronic pelvic inflammatory disease with obstructed tubes.

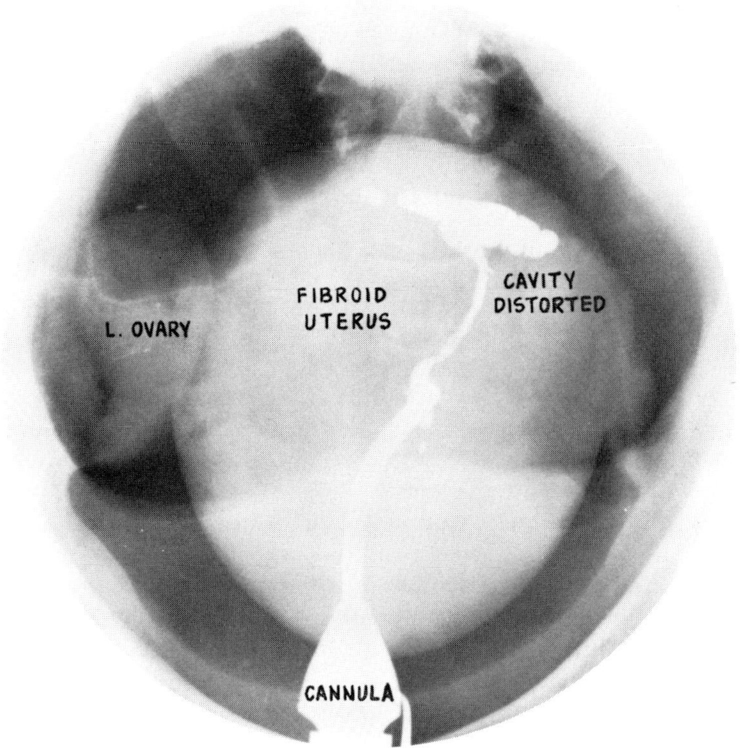


*Figure 16–7.* Large uterine fibroid shown by complete gynecography. Myomectomy restored fertility.

sorbed quickly. Slow introduction of gas will not accomplish the pneumoperitoneum necessary for adequate silhouetting of the intrapelvic organs.

9. Iodized oil,* approximately 5 ml., warmed to body temperature, is now instilled through the self-retaining cannula and the second film obtained.
10. The patient is rotated once again and the third film obtained in the dorsal position. Additional films may be taken for proper documentation of the hysterosalpingography.
11. The instruments are removed and the patient allowed to rest for approximately one hour until the effects of the narcotic have abated. Patients recover from this instrumentation very promptly, although some do complain of shoulder pain for a day or two.
12. A 24-hour spill picture may be obtained when tubal

*Lipiodol, Fougera and Co., Hicksville, Long Island, N.Y.

patency is in doubt. Table 16–1 gives the approximate x-ray exposure settings, depending upon the patient's weight and body configuration. Figures 16–4, 16–5, 16–6, and 16–7 show representative examples of studies obtained by this technique.

## INDICATIONS

Gynecography is indicated chiefly for obscure pelvic pathological conditions in which the usual methods of examination are inconclusive. Hence as a diagnostic technique it is complementary to culdoscopy and laparoscopy. At the Fertility Institute it is utilized to document the size and configuration of ovarian enlargements and as a feasibility study prior to myomectomy. We prefer complete gynecography to simple hysterosalpingography because more precise information is obtained.

Stein used this technique even for the differential diagnosis of unruptured ectopic pregnancy and early intra-uterine pregnancy. Should a pregnancy complication be suspected, tubal patency techniques would be contraindicated. Under these circumstances, pneumoperitoneum should be performed transabdominally. Stein utilized a short beveled 18-gauge spinal needle, approximately 8 cm. in length, inserted to the left and above the umbilicus. Stein did not use the Verres needle. The needle is inserted boldly through the skin and fascia, but cautiously through the peritoneum, and directed at a 45° angle down toward the pelvis. Frequently the abdominal wall is elevated with the left hand while the needle is advanced with the right hand. With experience it is possible to feel the needle penetrate each layer of the abdominal wall and the sudden "give" when the peritoneal cavity is entered. After the needle is inserted, approximately 1000 cc. of carbon dioxide is injected; this usually takes from one to two minutes. The patient is then rotated to a prone orientation and placed in a modified knee-chest position with the back arched; a film is obtained. Carbon dioxide gas is rapidly absorbed so evacuation of the pneumoperitoneum is unnecessary.

## CONTRAINDICATIONS

Transuterine pneumoperitoneum and hysterosalpingography are contraindicated in the following:

1. Suspected pregnancy complications.
2. Uterine bleeding.
3. Vaginitis and cervicitis.
4. Vaginal anomalies.

5. Acute or subacute pelvic inflammatory disease. (We advise routine white blood count and differential and erythrocyte sedimentation rates prior to gynecography.)
6. Pelvic tumors large enough to fill the true pelvis.
7. Cardiovascular or severe pulmonary disease.

Gynecography is best performed postmenstrually prior to ovulation. During amenorrhea, for example, in the diagnosis of Stein-Leventhal syndrome, one must make sure the patient does not have an early pregnancy.

## COMMENT

Kelling, one of the founders of laparoscopy, demonstrated the performance of air pneumoperitoneum in the dog in 1901, and many of the early laparoscopists, after employing pneumoperitoneum, obtained x-ray visualization of abdominal and pelvic organs. Goetze (1918) reported pneumoperitoneum for roentgen diagnosis as a new method. Orndoff, a roentgenologist in Chicago, in 1920 used this technique in association with the peritoneoscope for diagnosis of diseases of the abdomen. Other enthusiasts of this technique include Stein and Stewart (1919), Alvarez (1921), Peterson (1921), Yung (1923), Heuser (1924), Williams (1953), and Strauss and Cohen (1955).

Although gynecography was not a new technique when Stein and Arens employed it in 1923, they established it as a routine hospital x-ray procedure for the diagnosis of obscure pelvic diseases, especially in the infertile female. In a report dated 1929 they reported their experience in 470 patients. In 150 of these, iodized oil was employed in combination with carbon dioxide gas. They reported neither accident nor untoward result in this series of patients. Further, in none of those operated upon subsequent to this procedure was there evidence of peritoneal irritation or inflammation.

Following my association with Dr. Stein, we have continued to employ this technique. Since 1935 we garnered a vast experience with gynecography and have found it useful and harmless. At the Fertility Institute we still use it almost routinely for both its diagnostic and therapeutic values.

*Chapter Seventeen*

# ATLAS

There is an old Chinese proverb to the effect that one picture is worth ten thousand words. This atlas represents black-and-white reproductions of a selected group of Ektachrome transparencies culled from many hundreds of slides. My camera is always available during endoscopy to record in color the appearance of the pelvic organs. This collection of 49 slides contains 11 photographs obtained during culdoscopy; the remainder were obtained during laparoscopy. The photographic technique employed is discussed in Chapters 11 and 12.

Photography via culdoscopy is more difficult than photography by laparoscopy, inasmuch as the culdoscope is so close to the pelvic organs that usually only small areas are available for photography. It is difficult to obtain the panoramic views so typical at laparoscopy.

I have included in the atlas panoramic views for orientation and to illustrate the appearance of the normal ovary during the pre- and postovulatory phases. Ovaries showing failure of ovulation at culdoscopy are depicted in Figure 17–6 and at laparoscopy in Figures 17–16, 17–17, and 17–18. Ovulation induced by Pergonal and Clomiphene are pictured in Figures 17–15 and 17–19, respectively. The differential diagnosis between ectopic pregnancy and threatened abortion is illustrated in Figures 17–11, 17–24, and 17–25.

Pelvic adhesions, which are impossible to diagnose except by laparotomy or endoscopy, may be very minimal, or they may be extensive enough to prevent identification of the pelvic organs. Adhesions following ovarian resection (Figures 17–20, 17–38, 17–39, and 17–40) and secondary to pelvic inflammatory disease (Figures 17–35, 17–36, and 17–37) are very commonly found. Cautery of fine adhesions (Figures 17–41, 17–42, and 17–43) and the technique of ovarian biopsy (Figure 17–45) are demonstrated.

Because leiomyomata are diagnosed easily by pelvic bimanual examination, endoscopy is usually unnecessary; nonetheless, subserous and small intramural fibroids were photographed (Figures 17–27 and 17–28). Endometriosis, so frequently associated with pelvic pain and unexplained infertility, is demonstrated in Figures 17–9, 17–10, 17–12, and 17–30 through 17–34. On gross inspection it would have been difficult to differentiate the benign teratoma shown in Figure 17–29 from the endometrial cyst of Figure 17–30. The correct diagnosis was obtained at laparotomy. A "second look" after myomectomy, salpingostomy, and ovarian resection is demonstrated in Figures 17–20, 17–40, and 17–44. Diagnosis of anomalies of the uterus is usually made by digital and x-ray examinations; Figure 17–46 illustrates the appearance of a double uterus at laparoscopy.

It is possible for the gynecologic laparoscopist to view upper abdominal organs as well. Hence the normal liver and gall bladder are illustrated in Figure 17–47. The appendix may be frequently visualized, and the appearance of a normal appendix is compared with an acute appendicitis in Figure 17–48 and 17–49, respectively. I have not yet obtained photographs of acute salpingitis, carcinoma, or tuberculosis of the pelvic organs. Figure 17–35 shows the result of a severe chronic pelvic inflammatory process. This patient gave a history of pulmonary histoplasmosis.

The publishers have duplicated the original Ektachrome slides from which this atlas was derived, since most hospitals, schools, and physicians' offices have projectors for 2 × 2 slides. This collection of slides is available from the publishers. It is hoped that they will stimulate the endoscopist to become an endoscopic photographer in order to obtain proper documentation of his own cases and also for teaching purposes. I would suggest that as each slide is projected, the corresponding labeled black-and-white reproduction be reviewed.

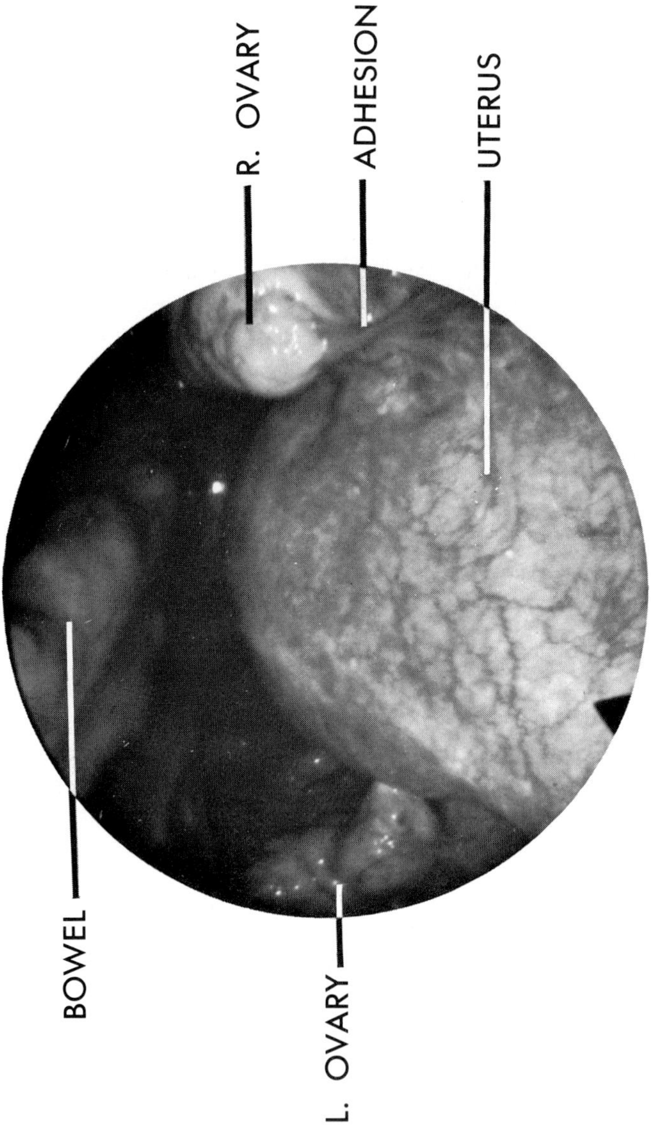


*Figure 17–1.* Panorama of uterus and adnexa at culdoscopy. Note minimal adnexal adhesions; bowel above.

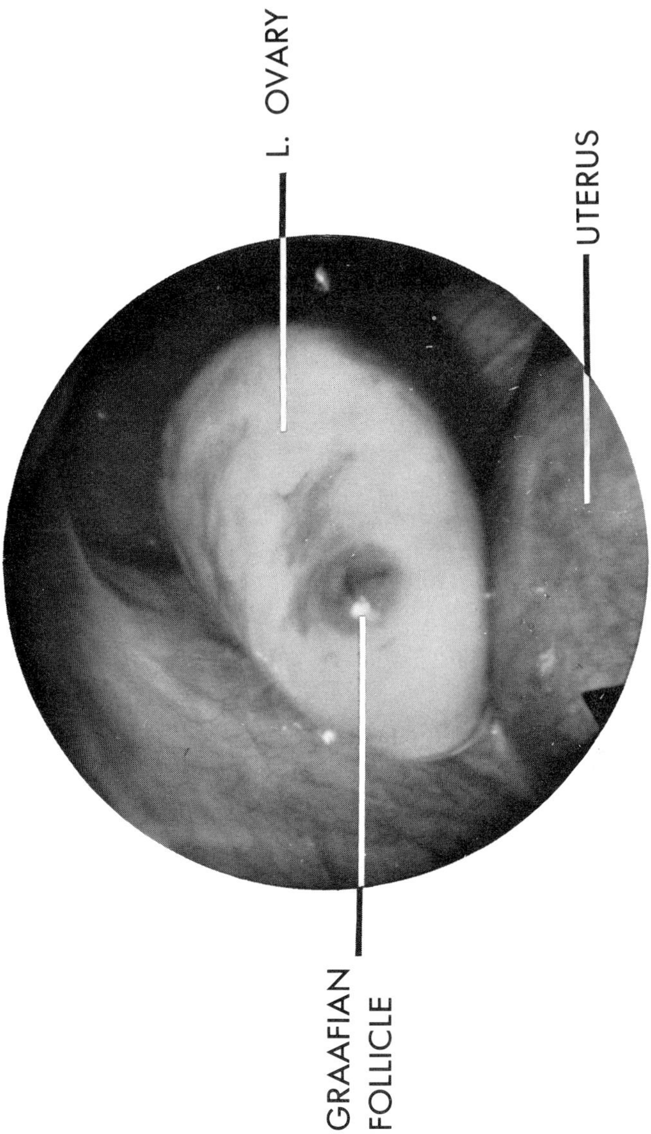


*Figure 17–2.* Culdoscopic view of normal ovary containing a superficial follicle with fine blood vessels on the surface suggestive of a Graafian follicle; uterus below.

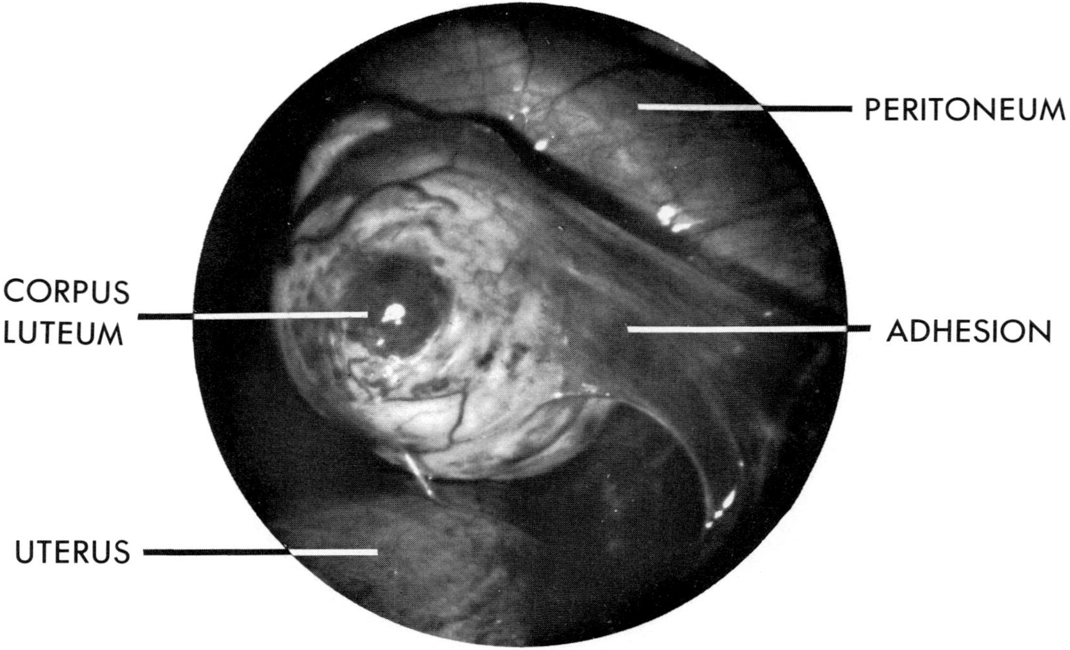


*Figure 17–3.* Culdoscopy. Ovary containing corpus luteum partially covered with a fine adhesion.

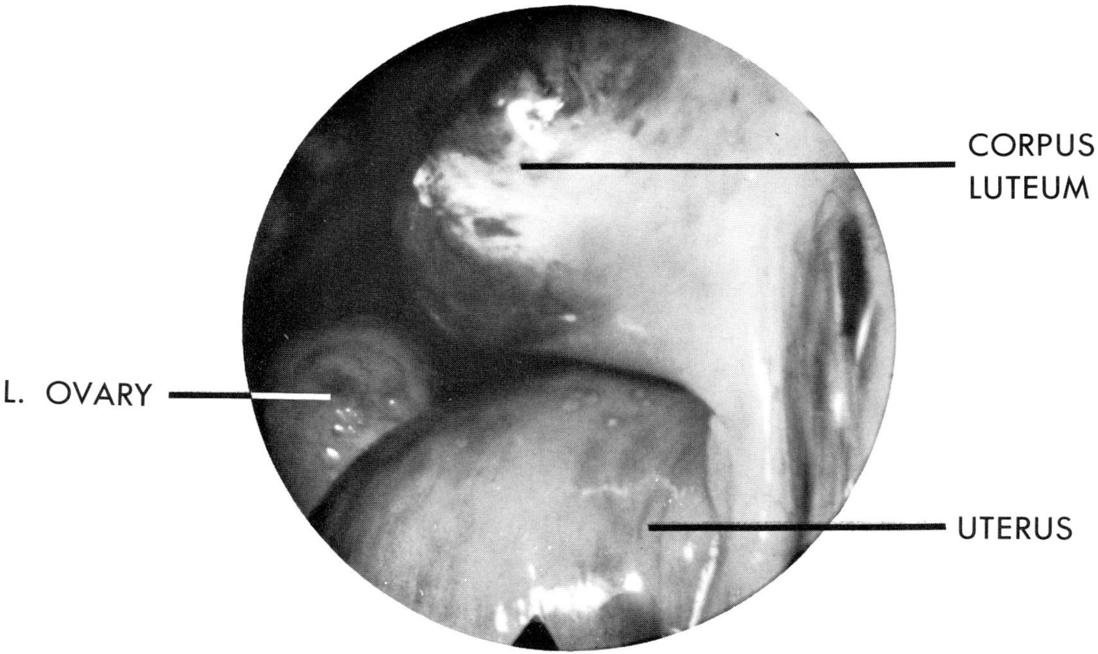


*Figure 17–4.* Culdoscopy. Panoramic view showing very vascular corpus luteum in right ovary. There is distortion in size of right ovary due to proximity to lens of culdoscope.

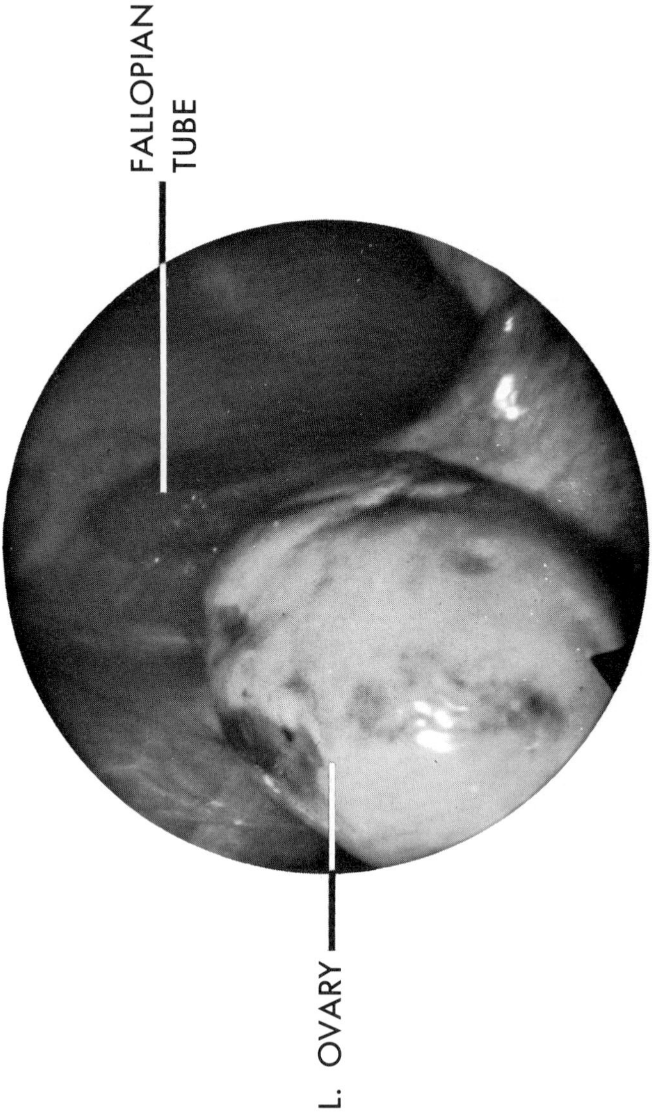


*Figure 17–5.* Culdoscopy. Normal left adnexa. The ovary contains a follicle cyst and an area of luteal tissue.

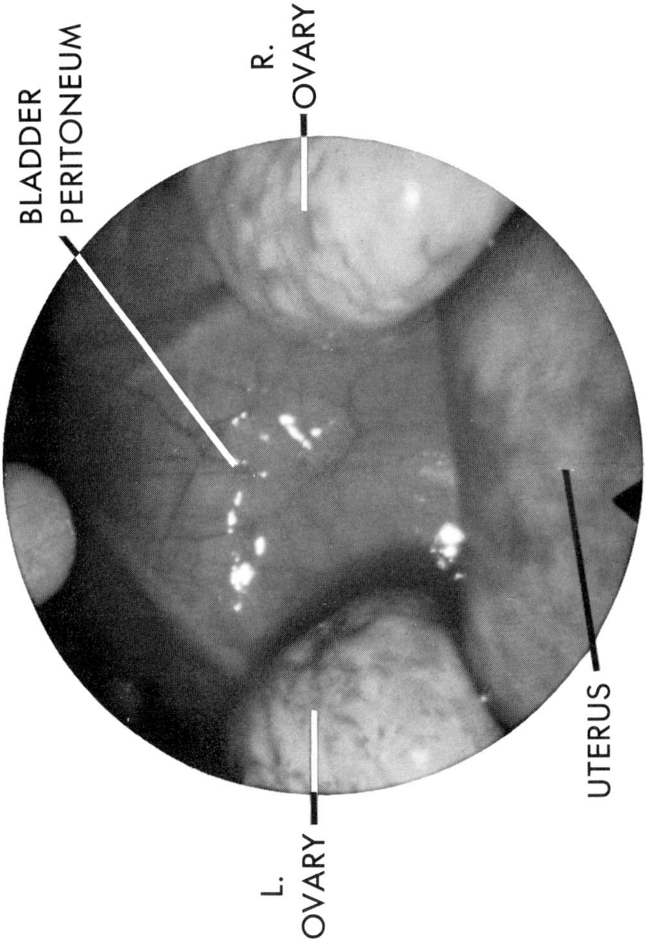


*Figure 17–6.* Culdoscopy. Typical bilateral polycystic ovaries.

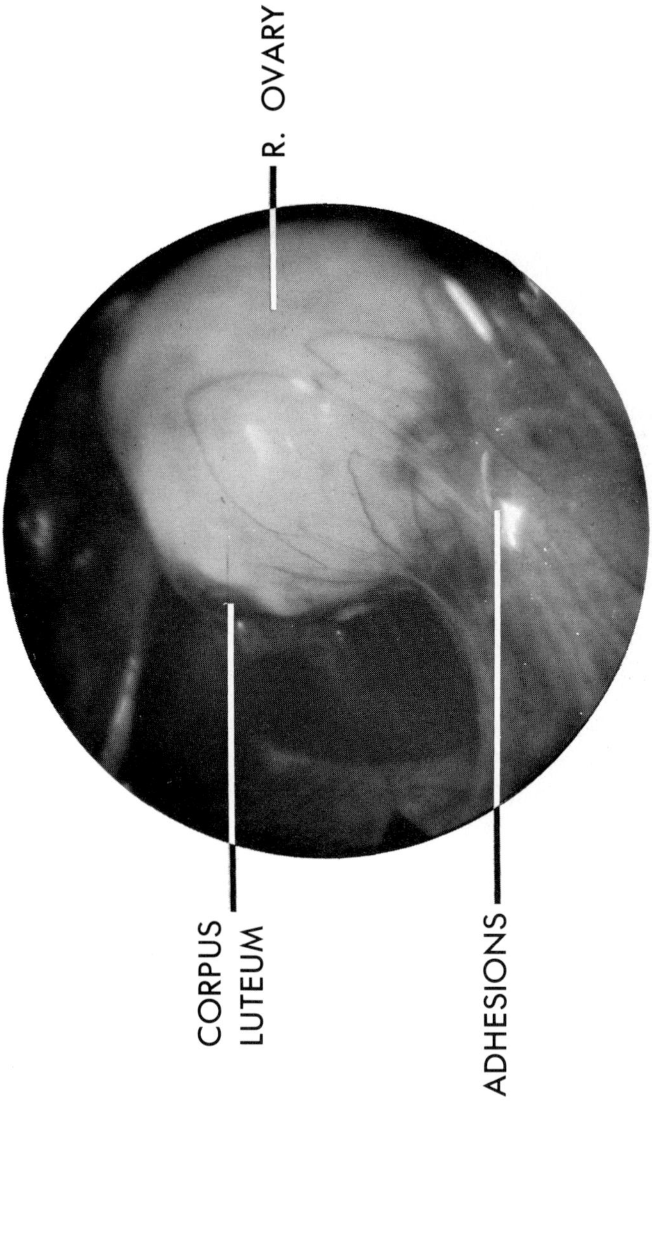


*Figure 17–7.* Culdoscopy. Ovary covered with fine adhesions. It is feasible to remove these adhesions with surgical diathermy at laparoscopy or operative culdoscopy.

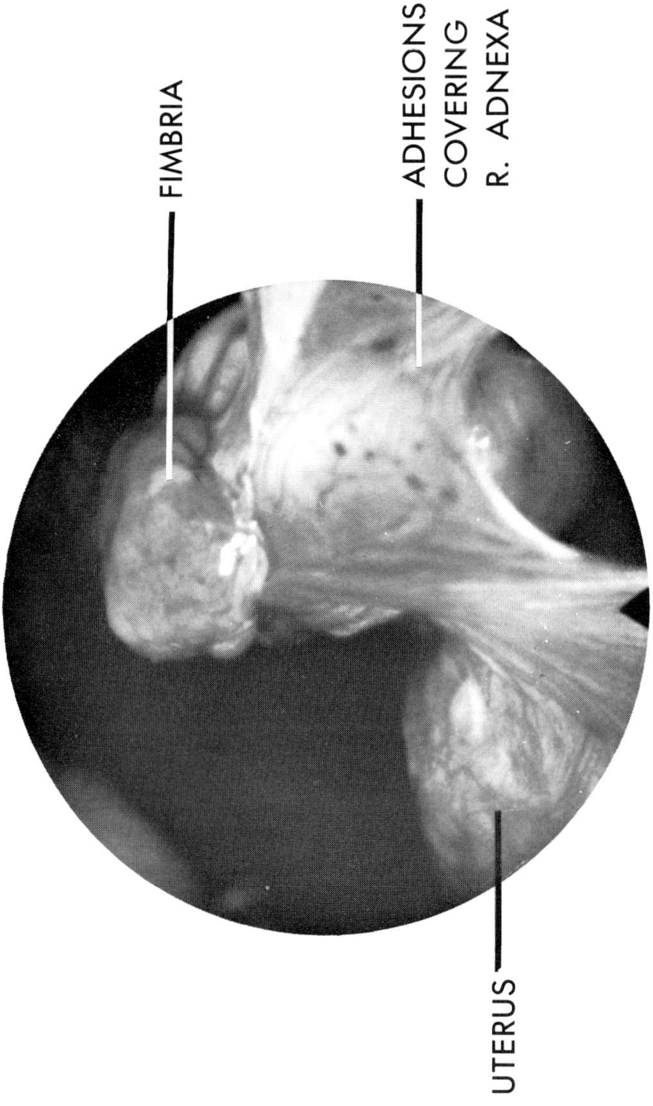


*Figure 17–8.* Culdoscopy. Right adnexal adhesions involving right ovary and uterus. The fimbria is free and normal.

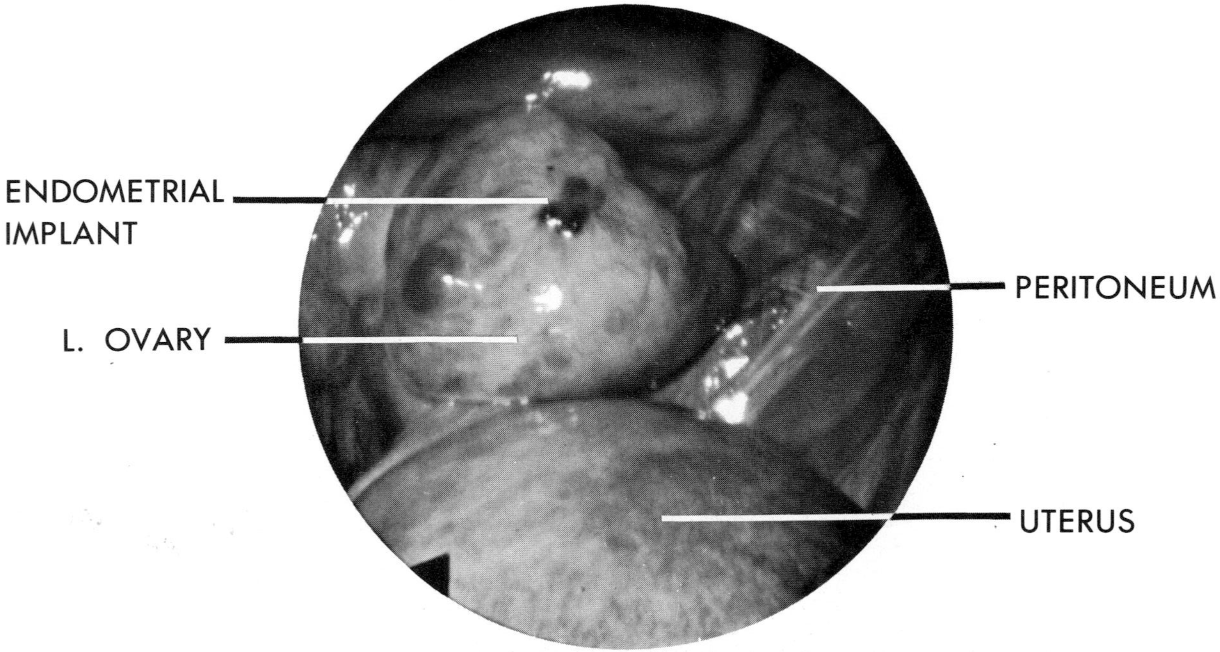


*Figure 17–9.* Culdoscopy. View of normal uterus below. Left cystic ovary contains a small endometrial implant.

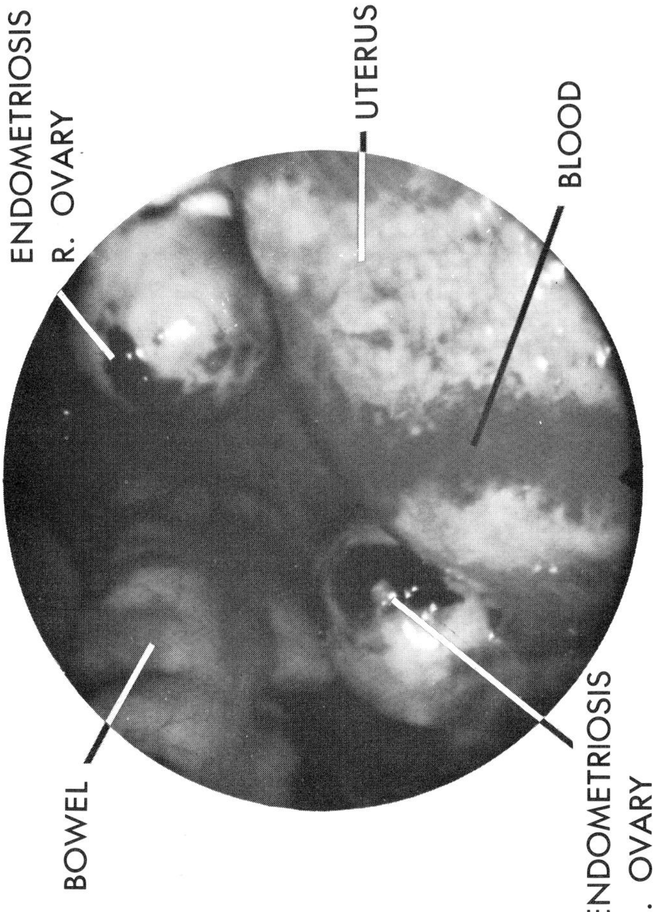


*Figure 17–10.* Culdoscopy. Endometriosis of both ovaries. Note uterus below with blood from puncture site.

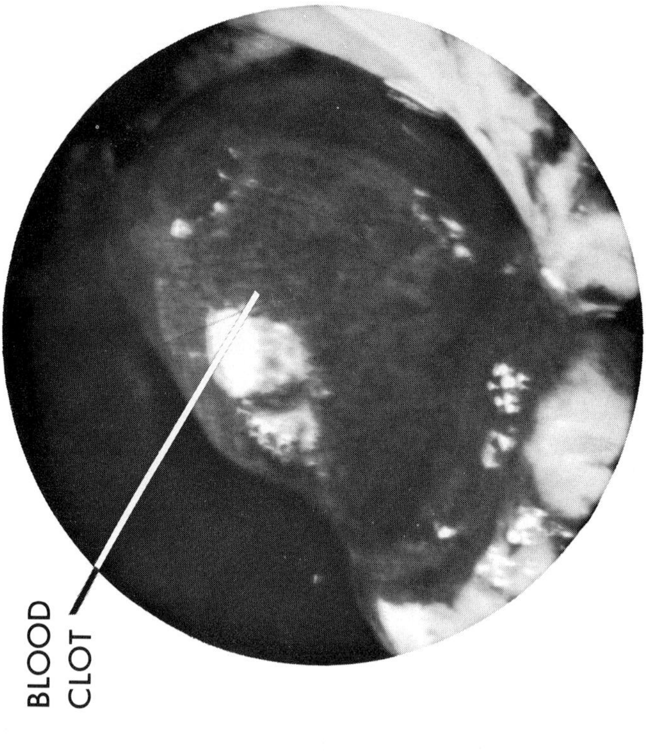


*Figure 17–11.* Culdoscopy. Blood clot from tubal pregnancy with tubal abortion.

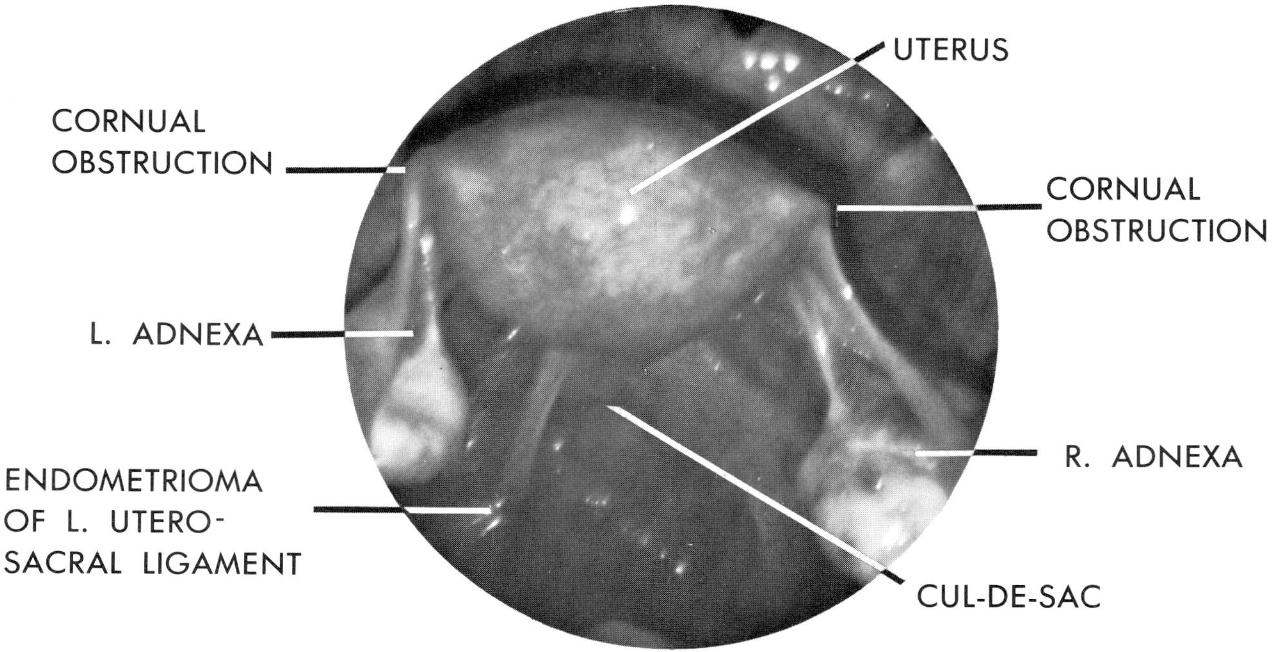


*Figure 17–12.* Laparoscopy. Prior hysterosalpingography in this infertile patient demonstrated cornual obstruction. Laparoscopy showed normal adnexa, but note the endometrial implant on the left uterosacral ligament. Our plan was progestogen suppressive therapy for possible isthmic endometriosis. Should conservative treatment be unsuccessful, this patient would be a candidate for tubal implantation.

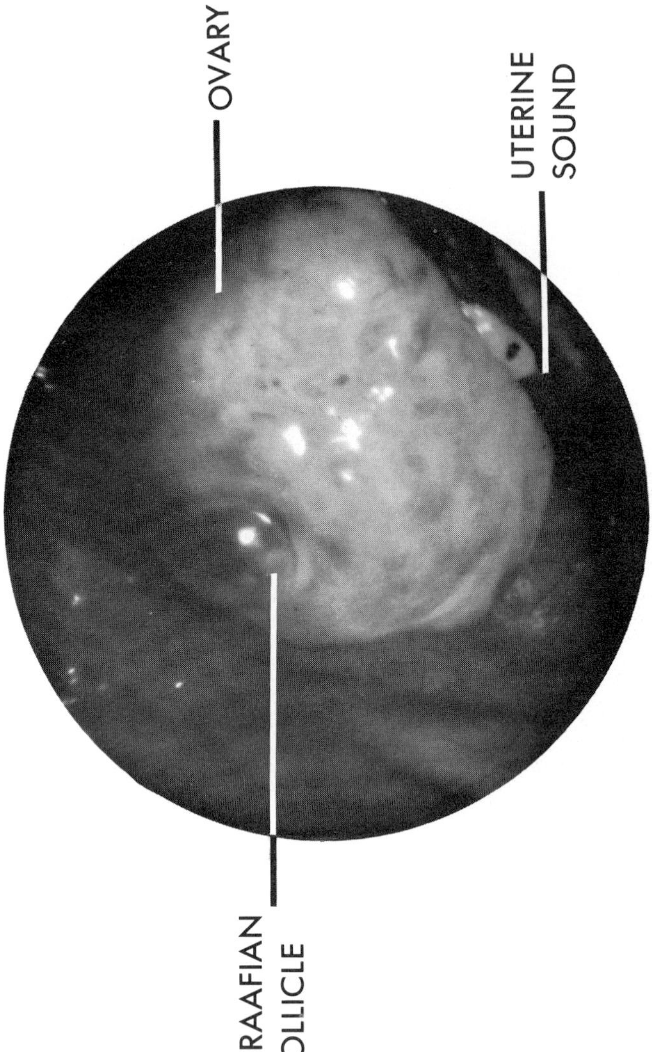


*Figure 17–13.* Graafian follicle at laparoscopy. Note uterine sound used as probe.

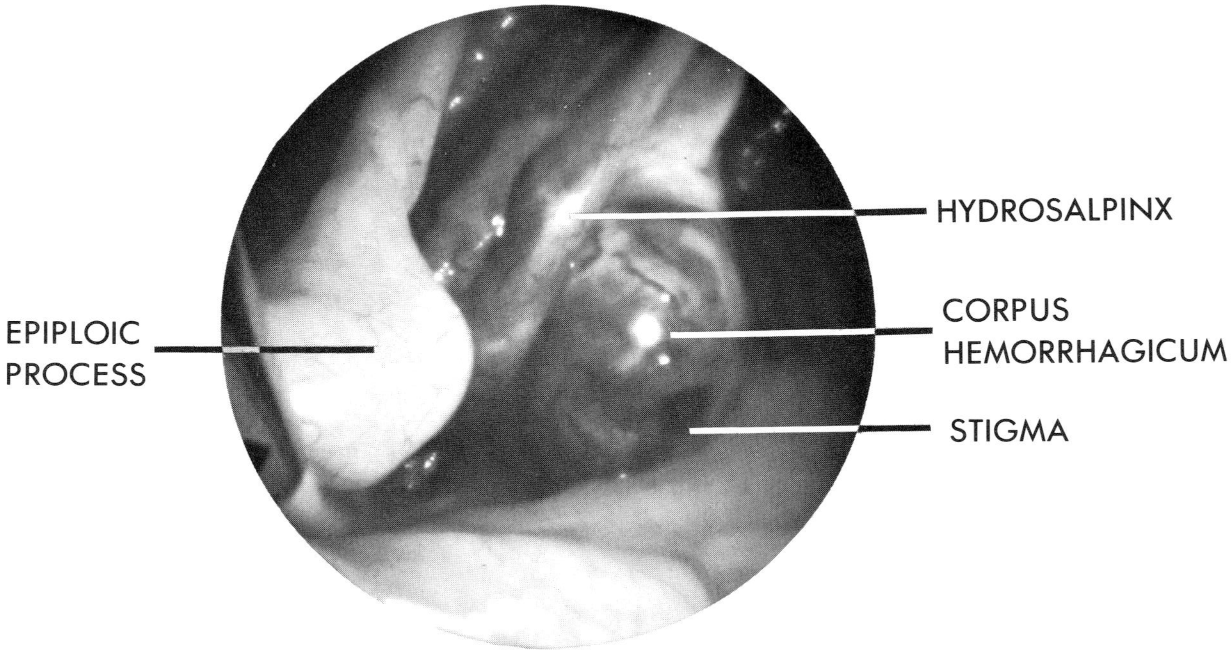


*Figure 17–14.* The detection of ovulation via laparoscopy is important. This is an early corpus luteum or corpus hemorrhagicum with a stigma. The hydrosalpinx was injected with indigo carmine dye. Lateral to the tube is an epiploic process.

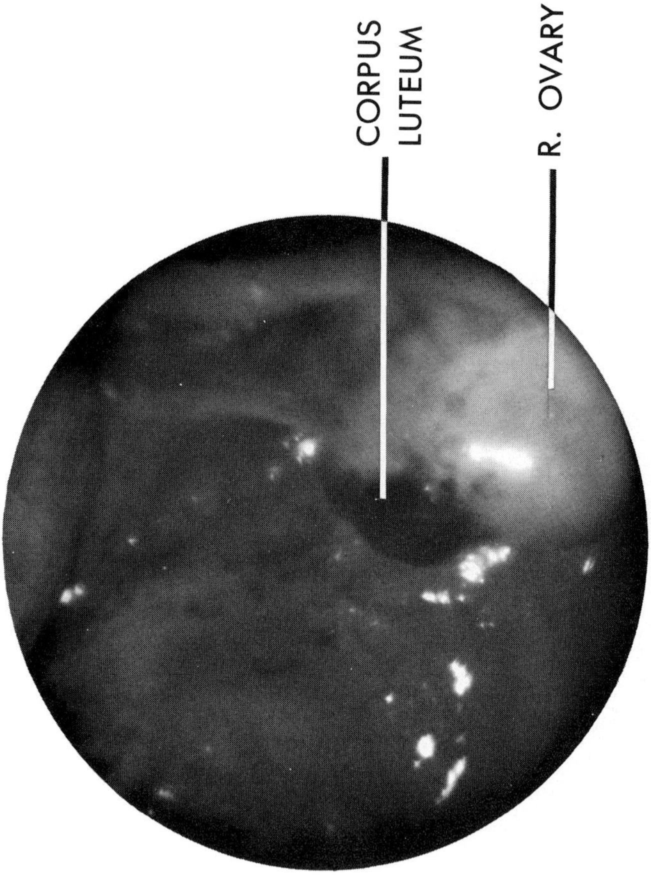


*Figure 17–15.* Laparoscopy. Corpus luteum induced by Pergonal (HMG) plus HCG. This induced ovulation resulted in pregnancy.

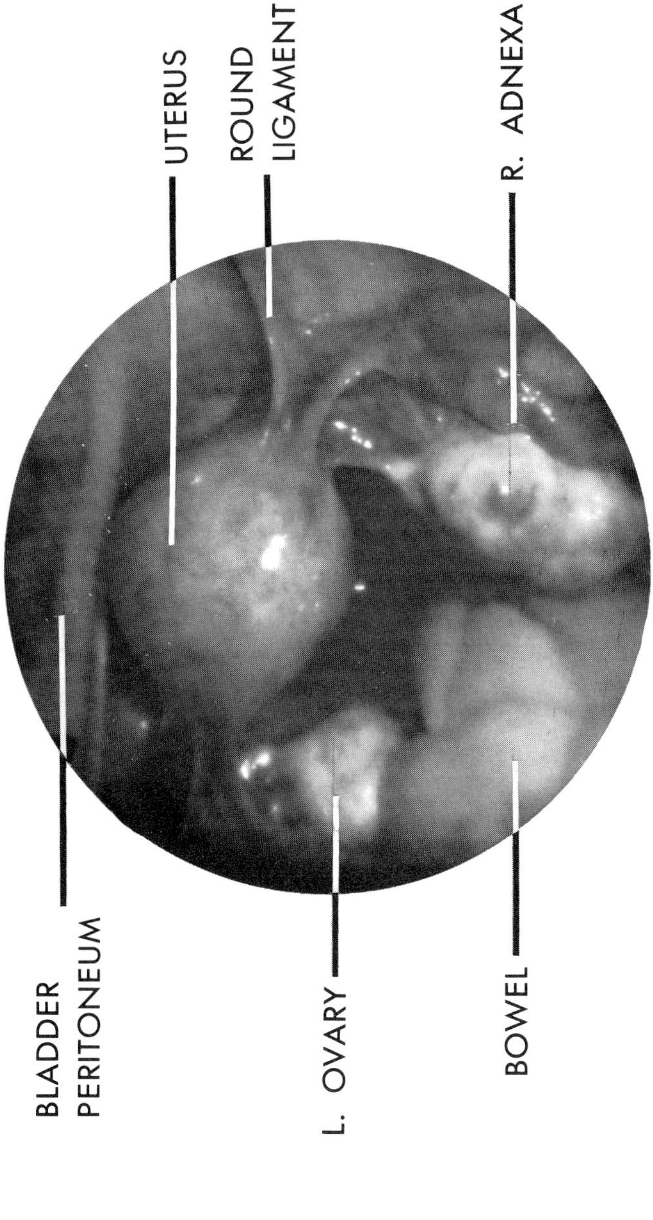


*Figure 17–16.* Laparoscopy. Panoramic view of patient with secondary amenorrhea. Note polycystic-type ovaries with very superficial follicles plus thin capsule.

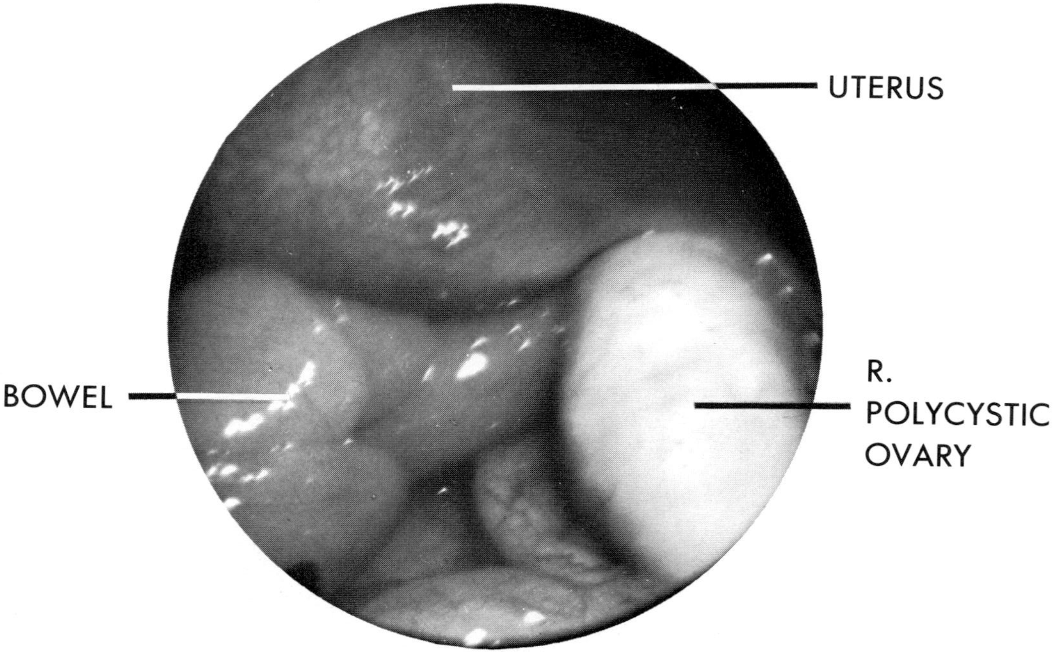


*Figure 17–17.* Laparoscopy. Uterus and right ovary in a patient with marked hirsutism and secondary amenorrhea.

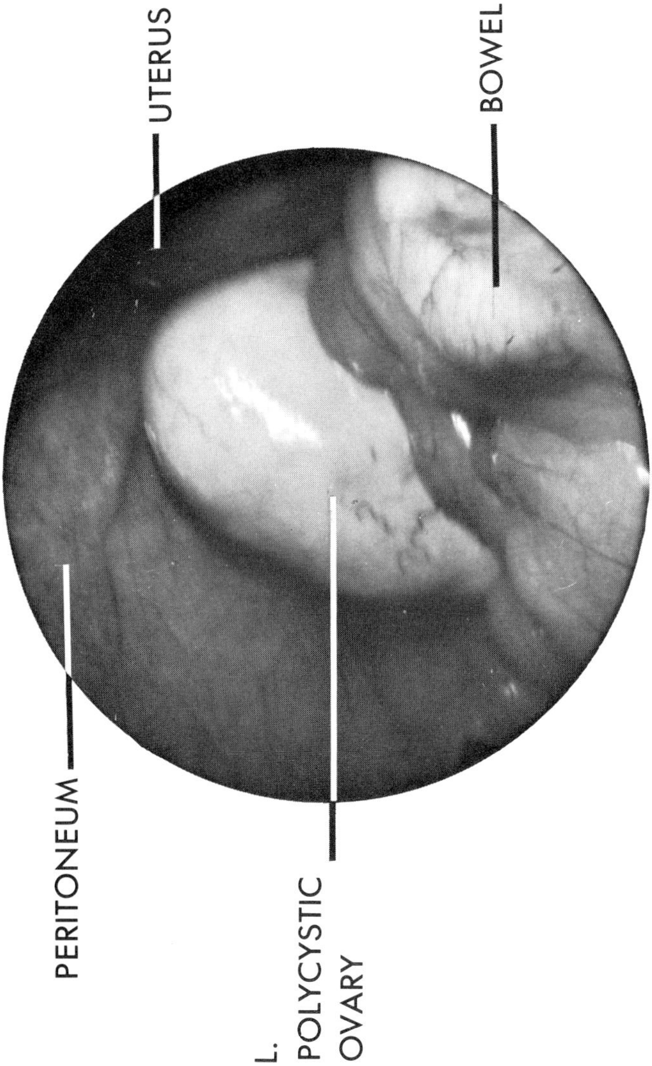


*Figure 17–18.* Laparoscopy. Left ovary of same patient as in Figure 17–17.

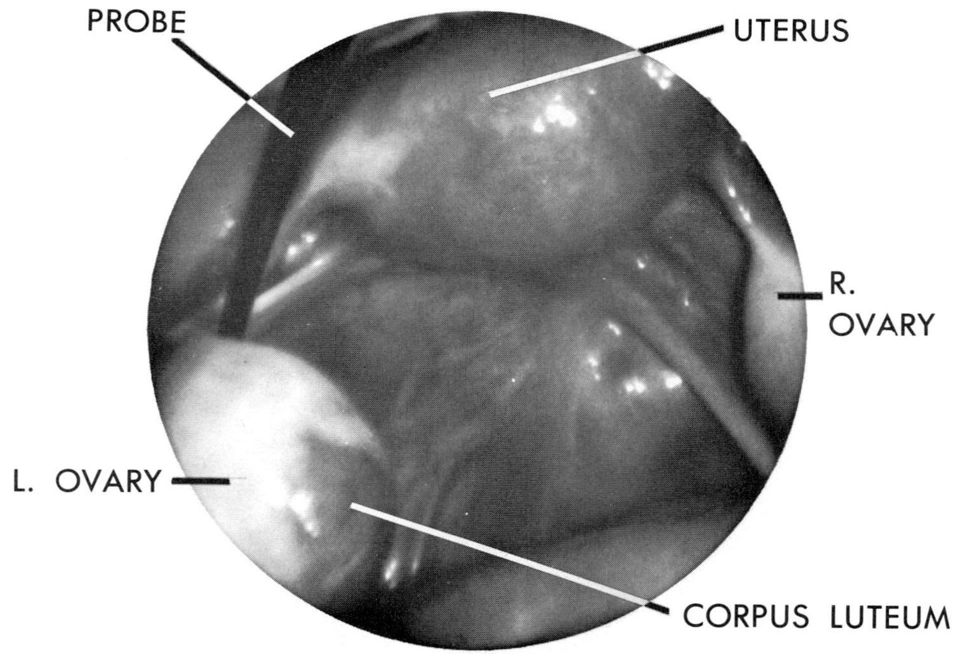


*Figure 17–19.* Laparoscopy. Patient with Stein-Leventhal syndrome with induction of ovulation in the left ovary following clomiphene citrate treatment. A normal pregnancy ensued.

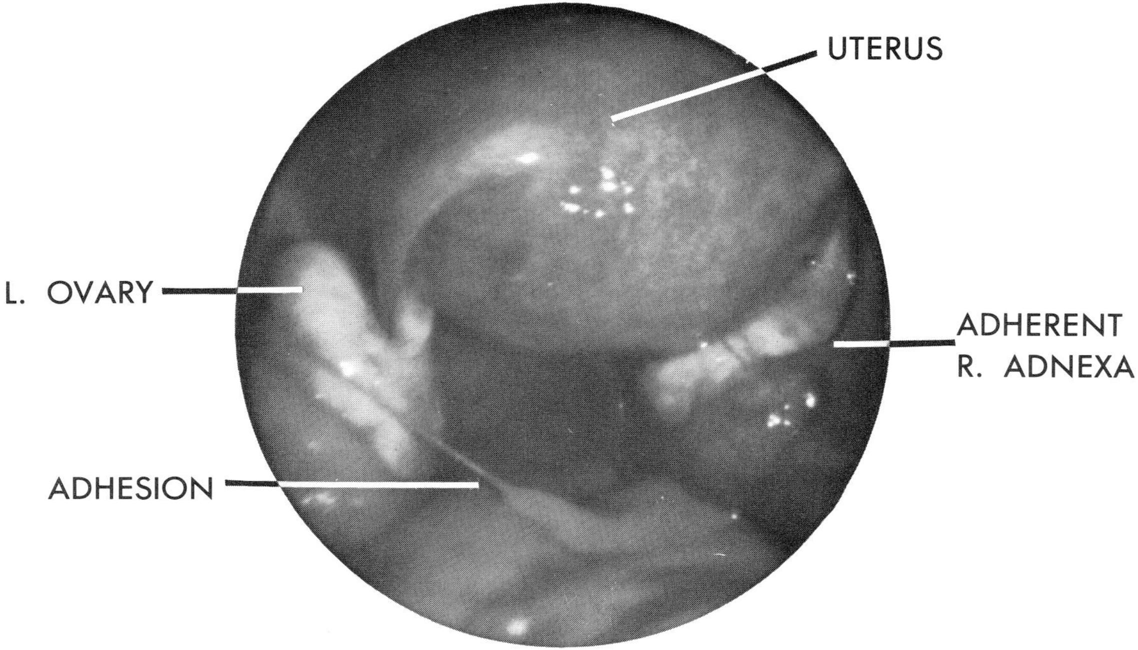


*Figure 17–20.* Laparoscopy. Bilateral wedge resection, performed six months prior to this laparoscopic examination. Although periods became regular and basal body temperature showed diphasic curves, the patient did not conceive. Semen and postcoital tests normal. Laparoscopy disclosed bilateral adnexal adhesions.

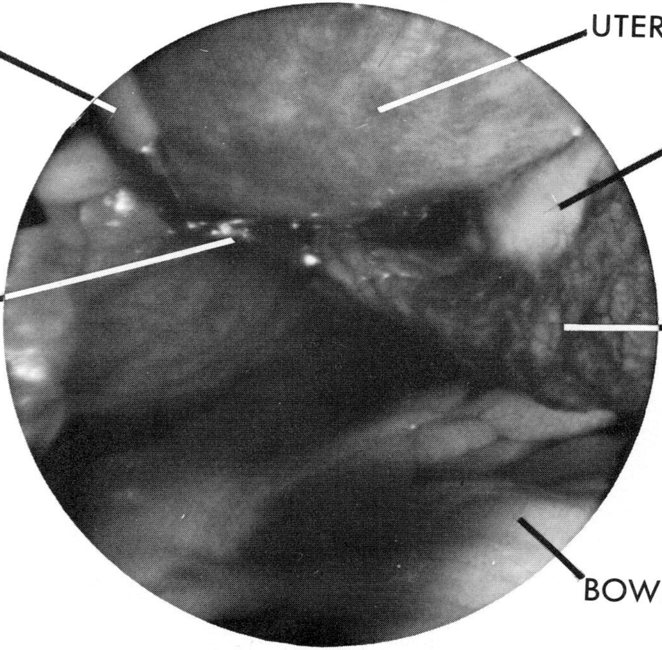


*Figure 17–21.* Laparoscopy. Same patient. Close-up of right adnexa with right fallopian tube distended with indigo carmine dye. Note how indigo carmine is trapped at fimbria; the right adnexa is adherent to the posterior leaf of the broad ligament. Adoption advised.

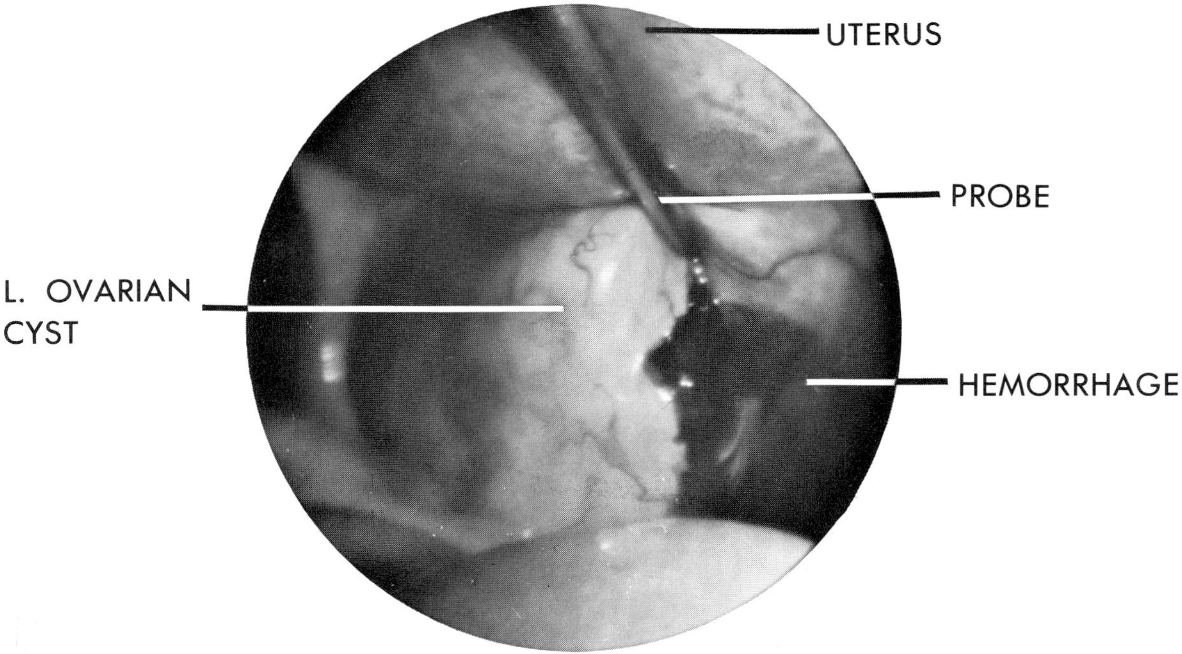


*Figure 17–22.* Laparoscopy. Probe used to dislodge this cul-de-sac cyst caused rupture of the capsule and hemorrhage. Corpus luteum cyst found at laparotomy.

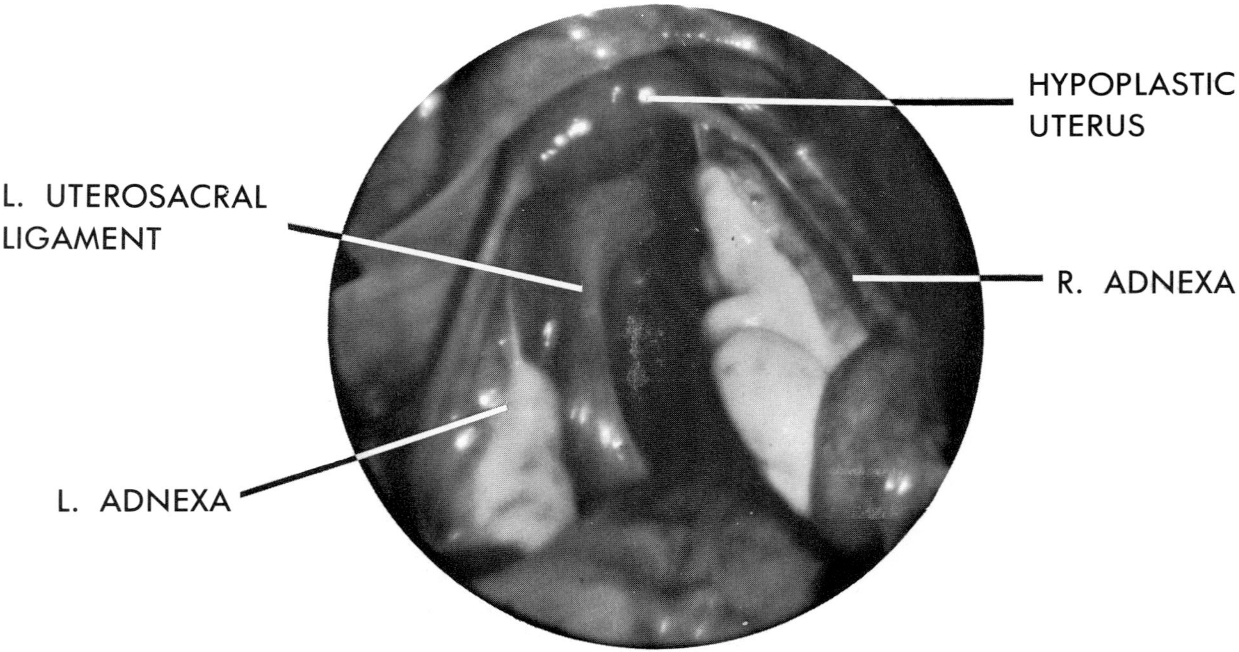


*Figure 17–23.* Laparoscopy has been extremely helpful in the classification of amenorrhea. In this 28-year-old patient with primary amenorrhea, laparoscopy demonstrated a hypoplastic uterus with elongated fallopian tubes and oysterlike ovaries with follicles.

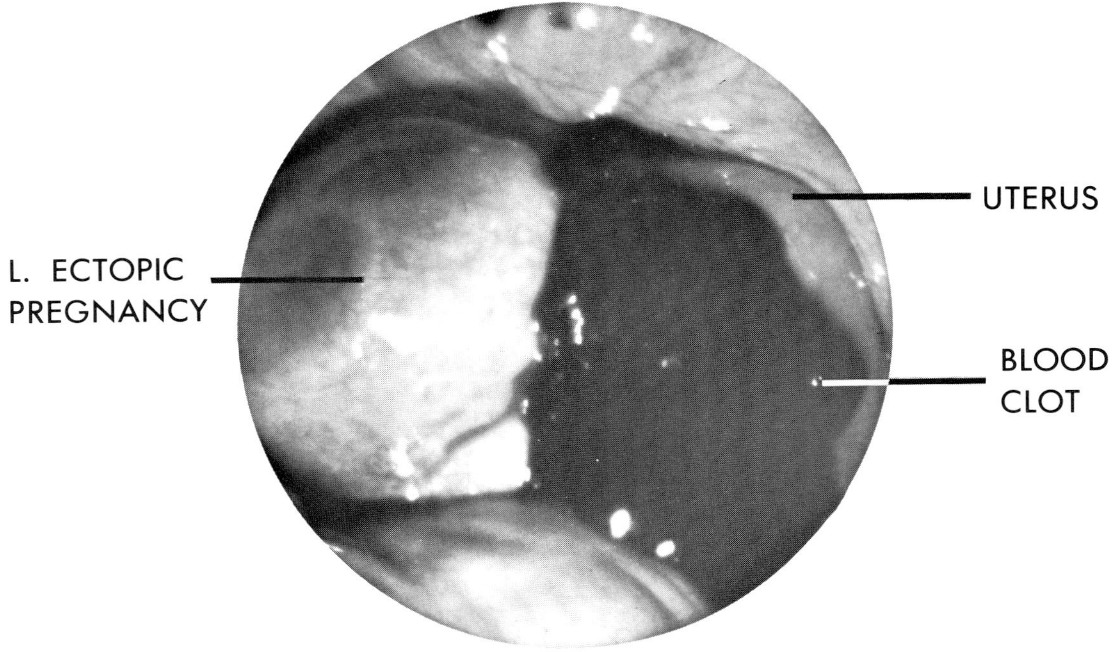


*Figure 17–24.* Laparoscopy has been an invaluable procedure for the diagnosis of unruptured tubal pregnancy. In this patient, beginning tubal abortion was present with a blood clot attached to a left tubal pregnancy.

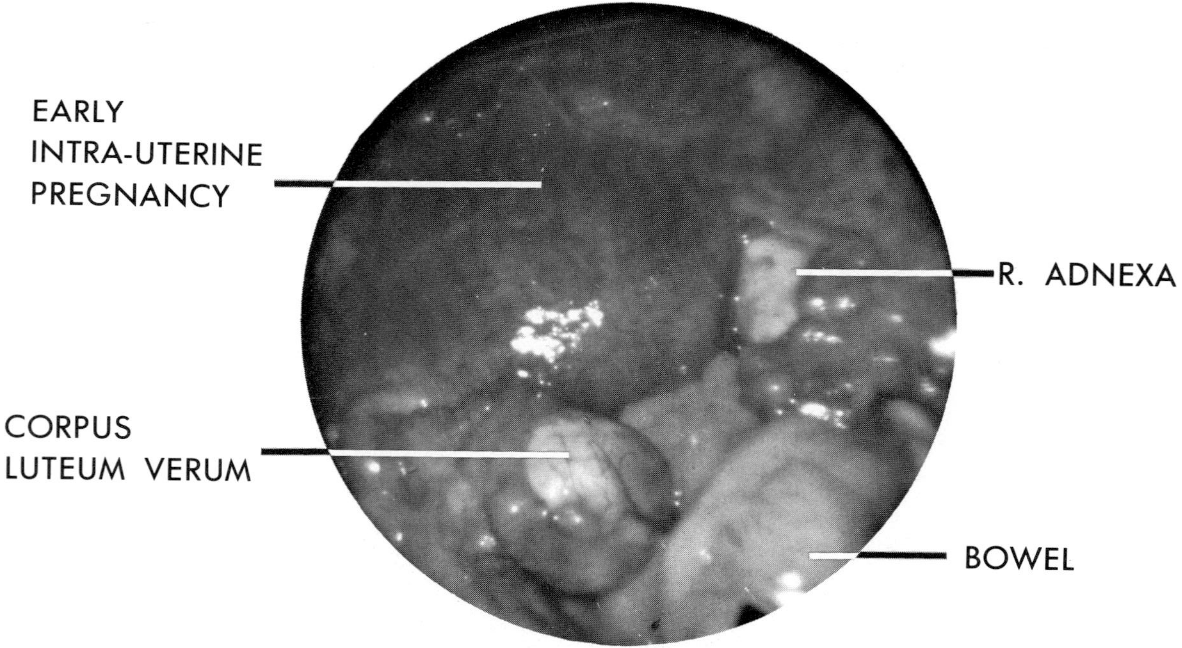


*Figure 17–25.* Laparoscopy. The preoperative diagnosis was suspected ectopic pregnancy; an early intra-uterine pregnancy was found. The mass detected on examination proved to be a left corpus luteum verum. This procedure does not disturb a normal pregnancy.

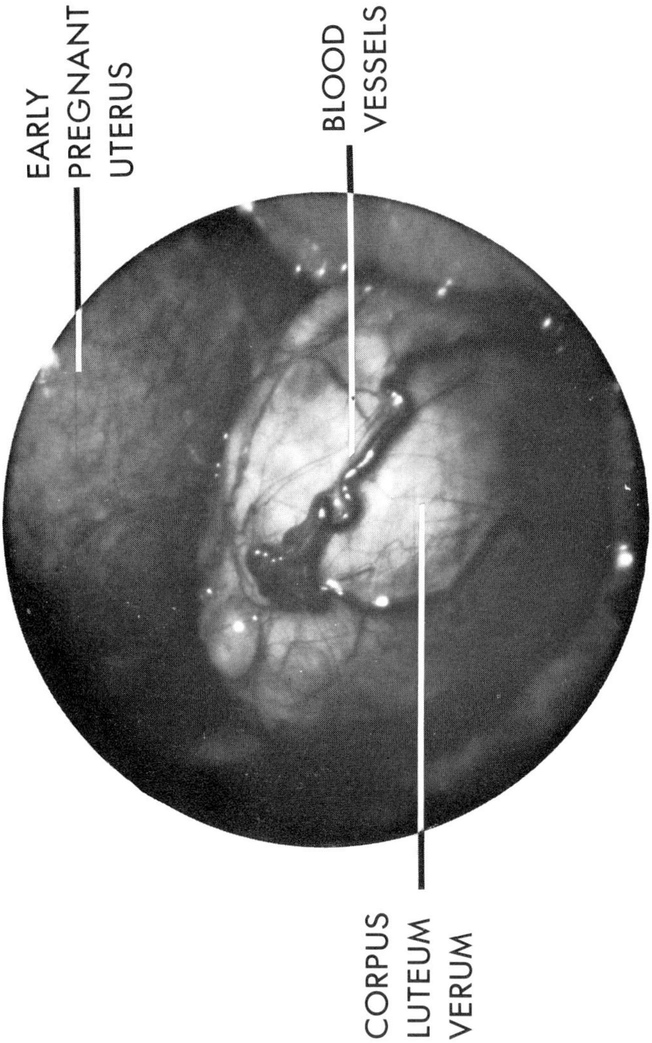


*Figure 17–26.* Laparoscopy. Same patient as in Figure 17–25. Close-up of corpus luteum verum with blood vessels coursing over surface.

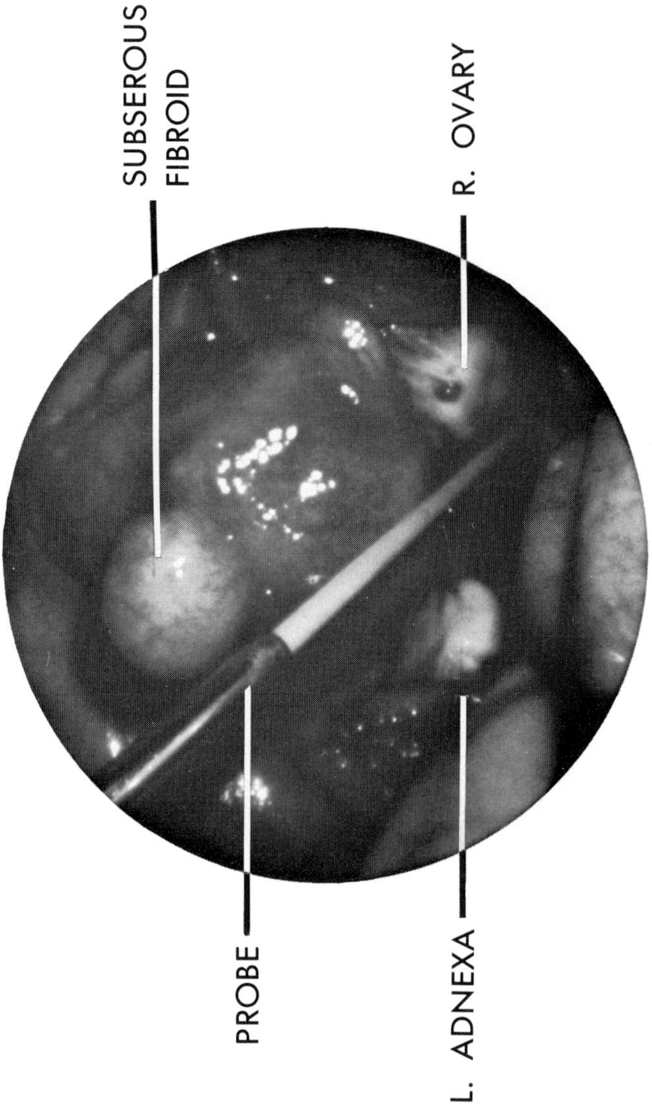


*Figure 17–27.* Laparoscopy. Large subserous fibroid; probe demonstrating normal adnexa.

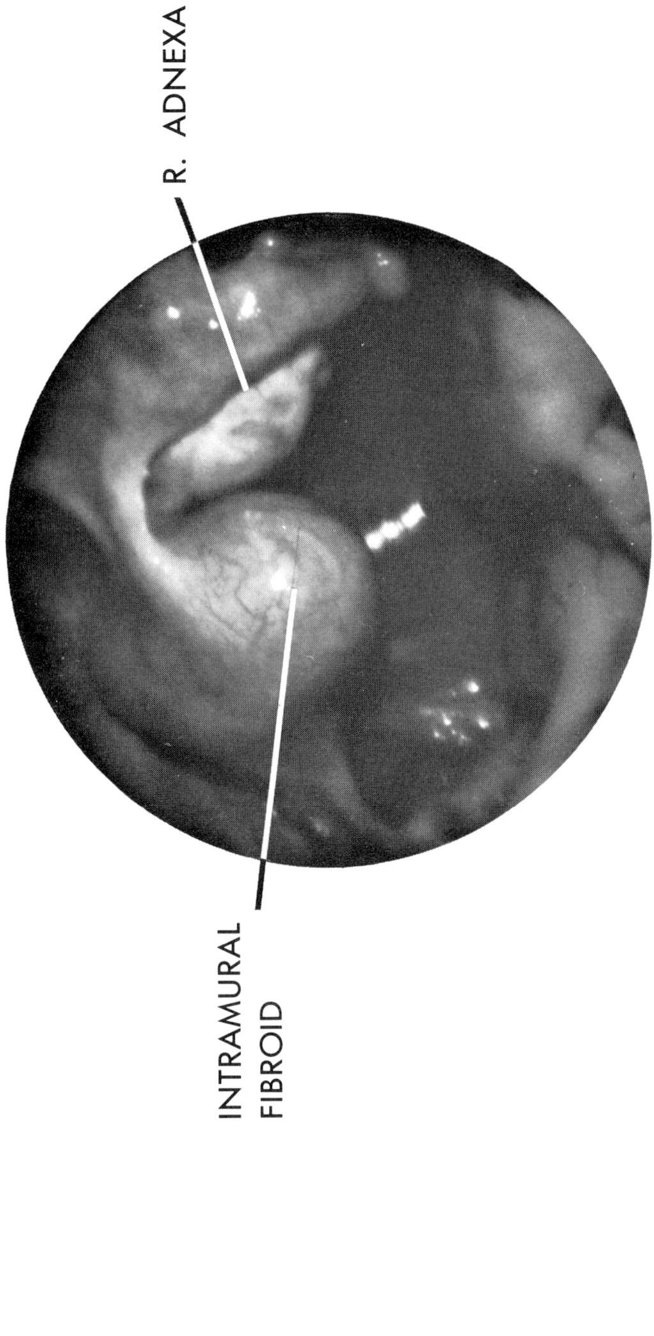


*Figure 17–28.* Laparoscopy. Intramural fibroid; normal right adnexa with positive tubal patency demonstrated with indigo carmine dye.

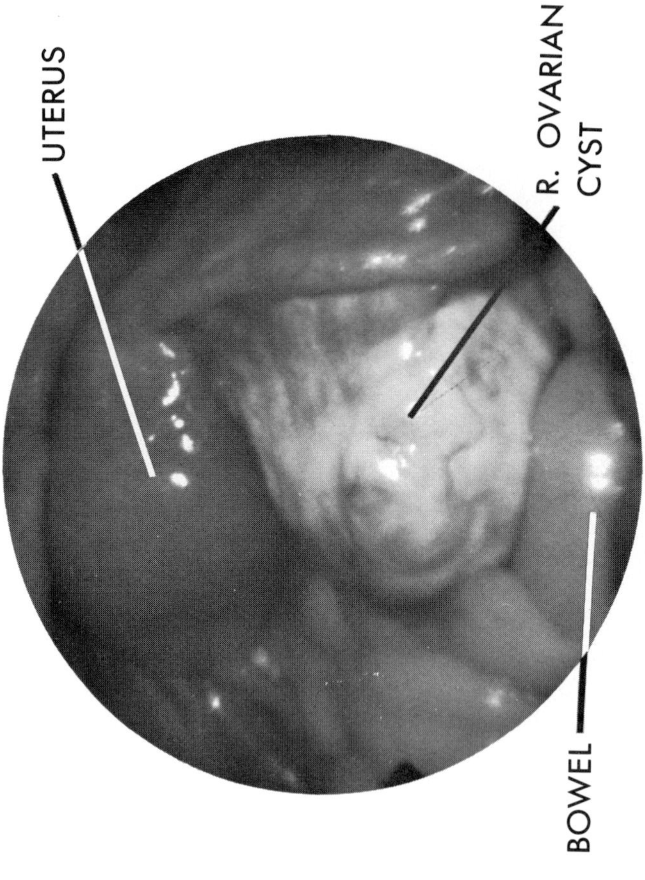


*Figure 17–29.* Laparoscopy. Panoramic view showing large ovarian cyst which proved to be a benign teratoma at laparotomy.

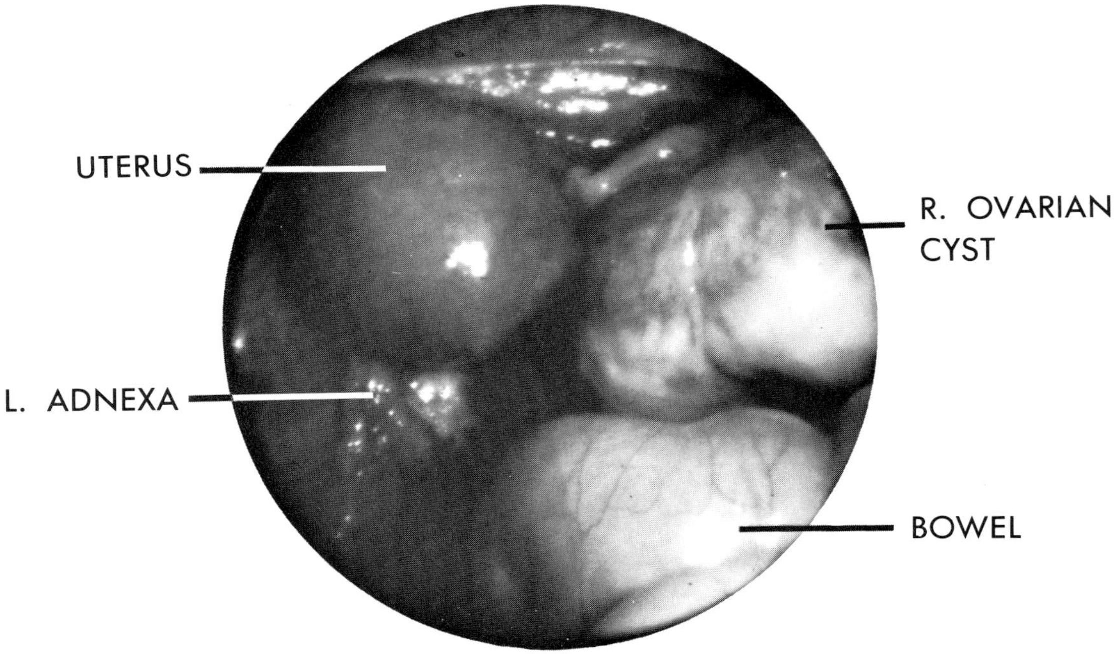


*Figure 17–30.* Laparoscopy. This infertile patient complained of pelvic pain. Laparoscopy disclosed a right ovarian mass which proved to be an endometrial cyst at laparotomy.

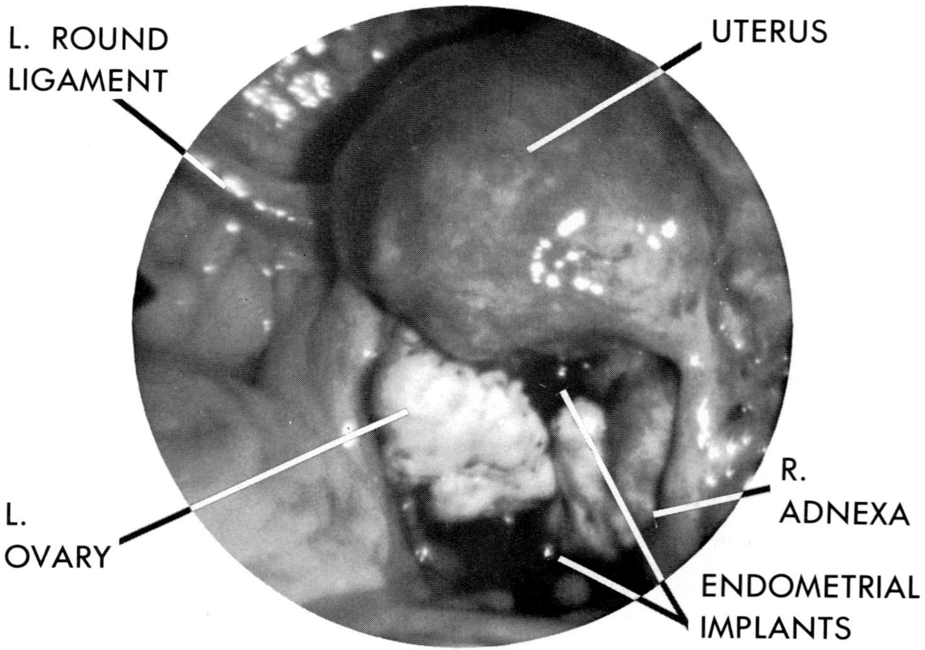


*Figure 17–31.* Laparoscopy. Pelvic examination on this infertile patient indicated an obscure cul-de-sac mass. Laparoscopy visualized both ovaries adherent to the utero-sacral ligaments with endometrial implants. Laparotomy was indicated.

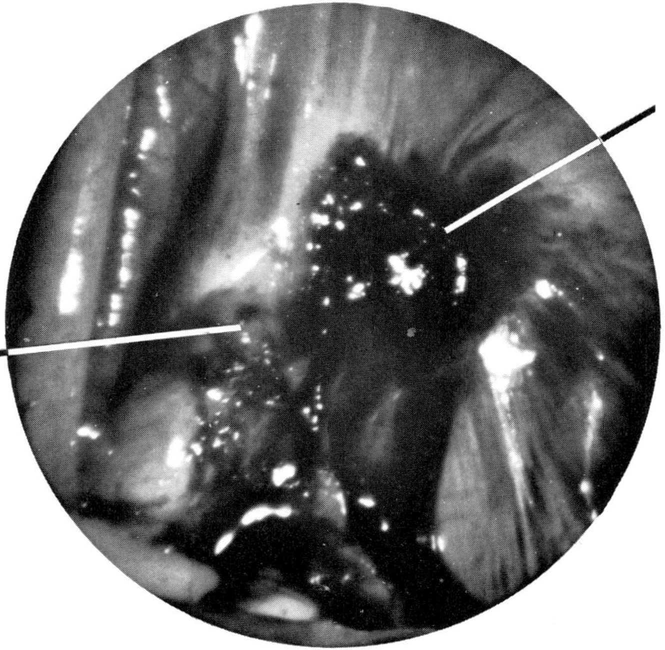


*Figure 17–32.* Cul-de-sac endometriosis in the process of high-frequency cauterization during laparoscopy.

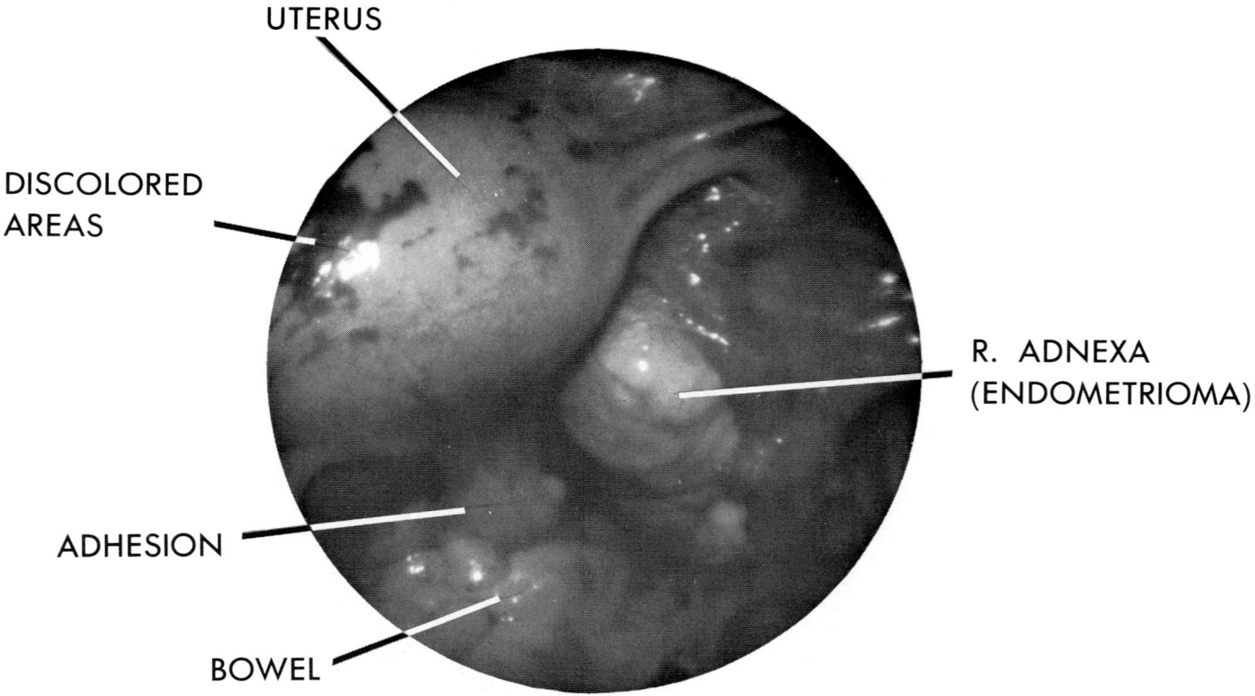


*Figure 17–33.* Laparoscopic view of pelvic structures showing uterus discolored with brownish substance suggestive of endometriosis. Bowel with adhesions obscures cul-de-sac. There is an endometrial cyst on right ovary.

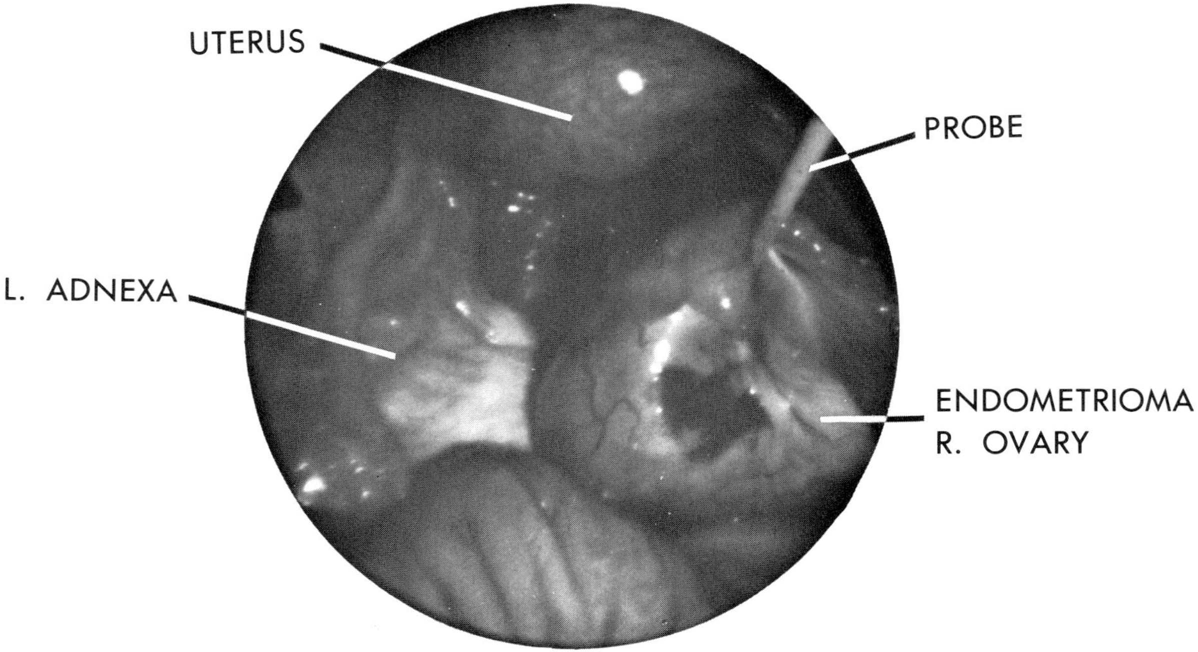


*Figure 17–34.* Laparoscopy. Panoramic view of pelvis showing probe elevating right adnexa. This right ovarian cyst containing an endometrioma would be more amenable to surgical intervention.

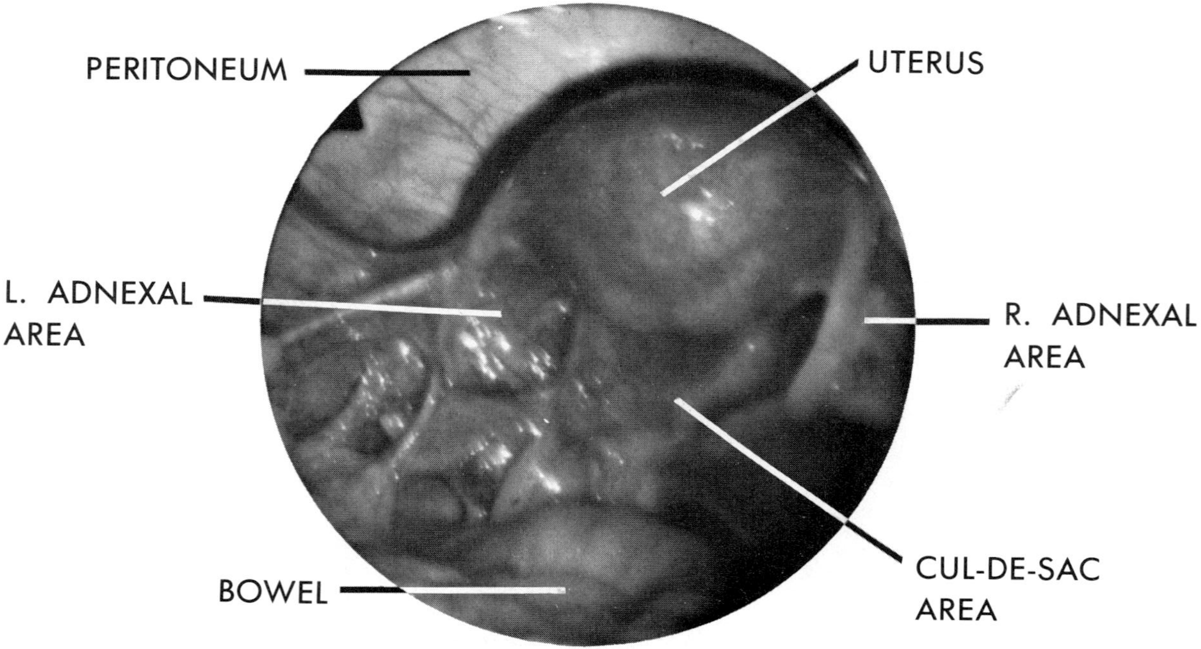


*Figure 17–35.* Laparoscopy. Pelvic inflammatory disease; adnexa impossible to identify. The patient had a history of pulmonary histoplasmosis.

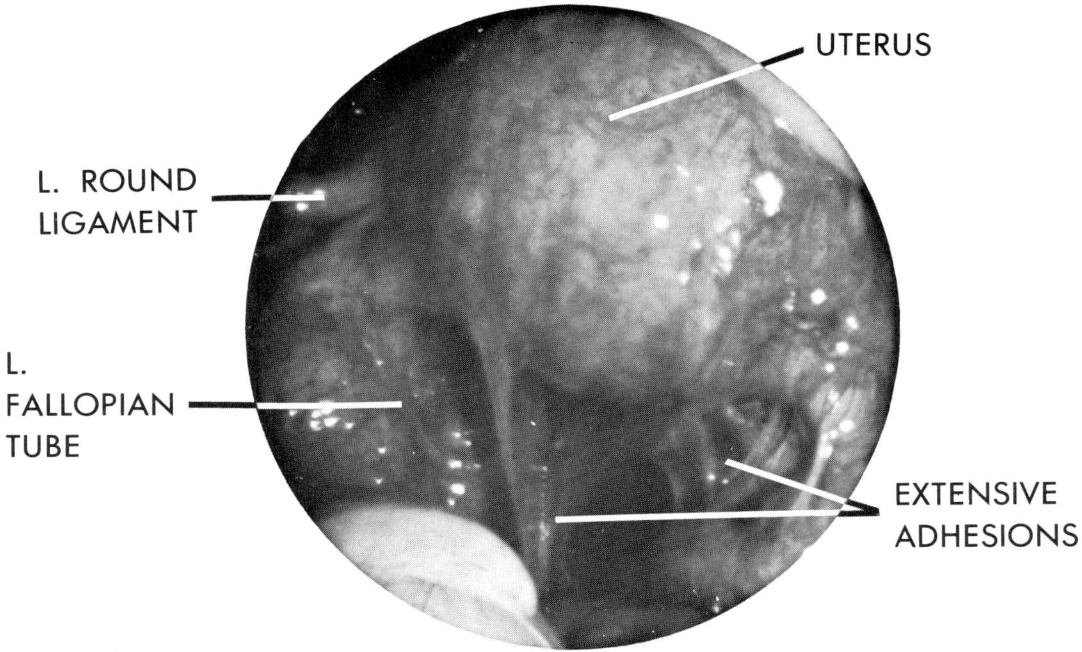


*Figure 17–36.* Laparoscopy. This infertile patient had extensive pelvic adhesions. We know of no other diagnostic technique that could demonstrate such a pathologic condition so beautifully. Laparotomy was performed with lysis of adhesions and salpingostomy.

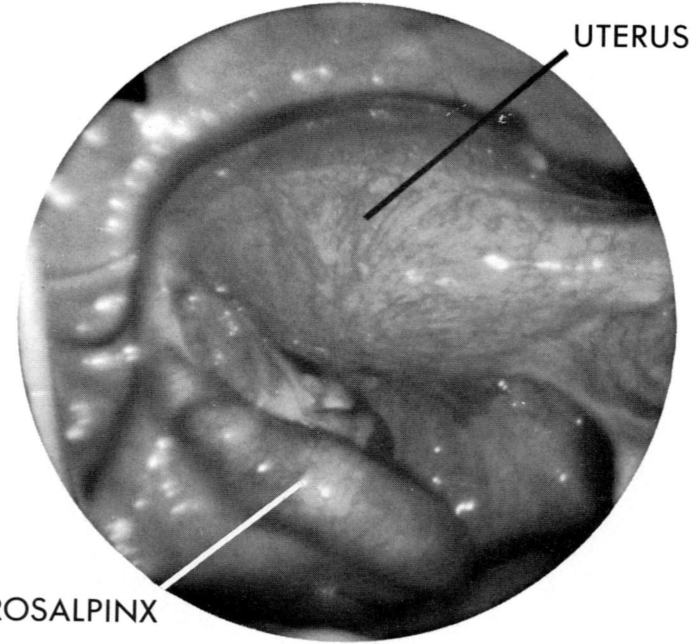


*Figure 17–37.* Laparoscopy. Left hydrosalpinx distended with indigo carmine dye. Culdoscopy was contraindicated, but hysterosalpingography would have been diagnostic.

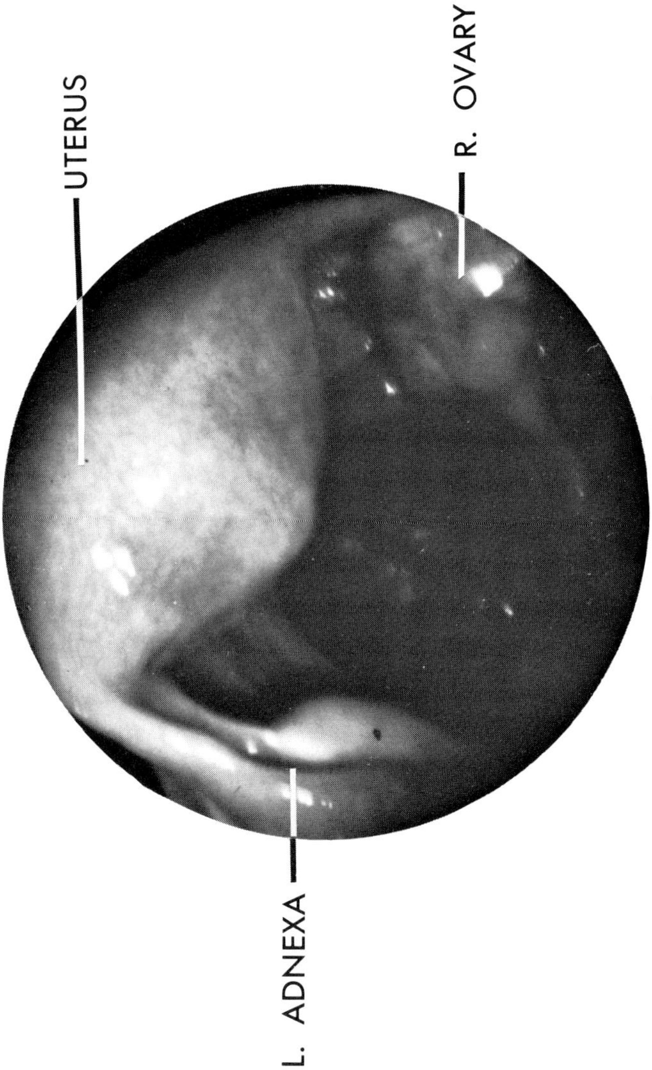


*Figure 17–38.* Panoramic view at laparoscopy. Prior right ovarian resection.

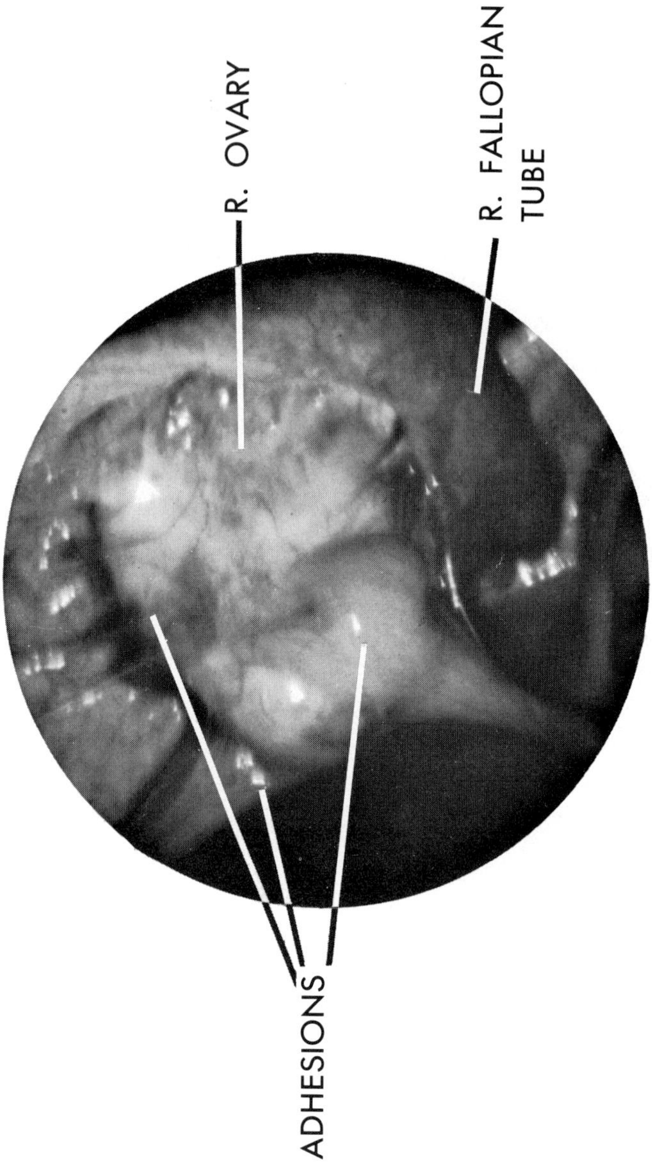


*Figure 17–39.* Laparoscopy. Same patient as in Figure 17–38. View showing adherent right ovary.

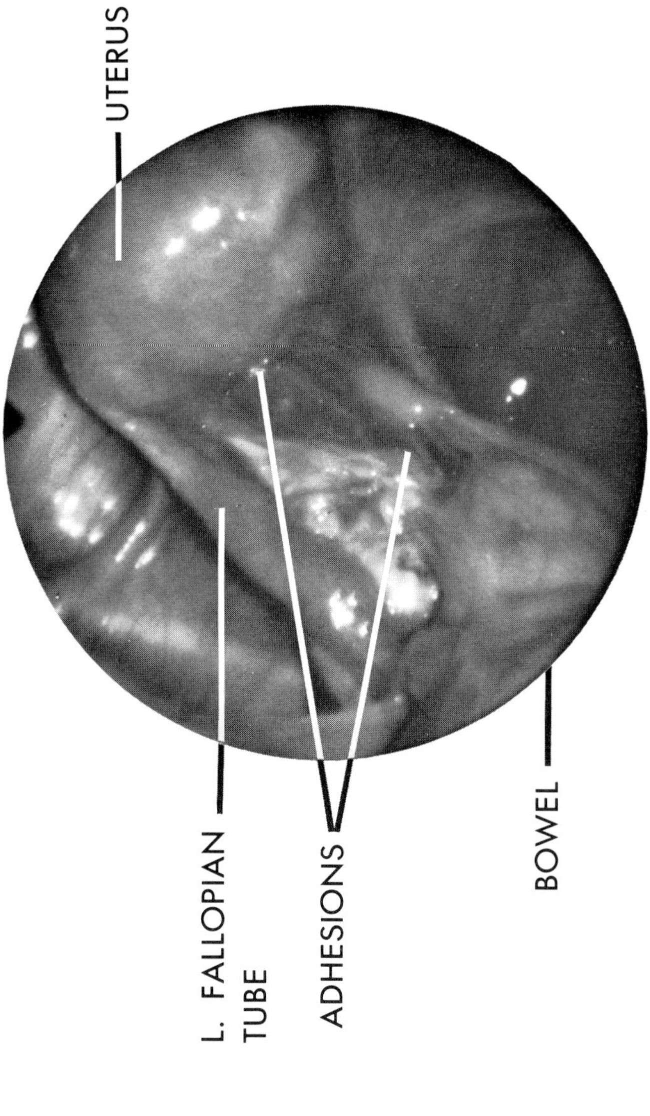


*Figure 17–40.* Laparoscopic view showing uterus with left adnexal adhesions.

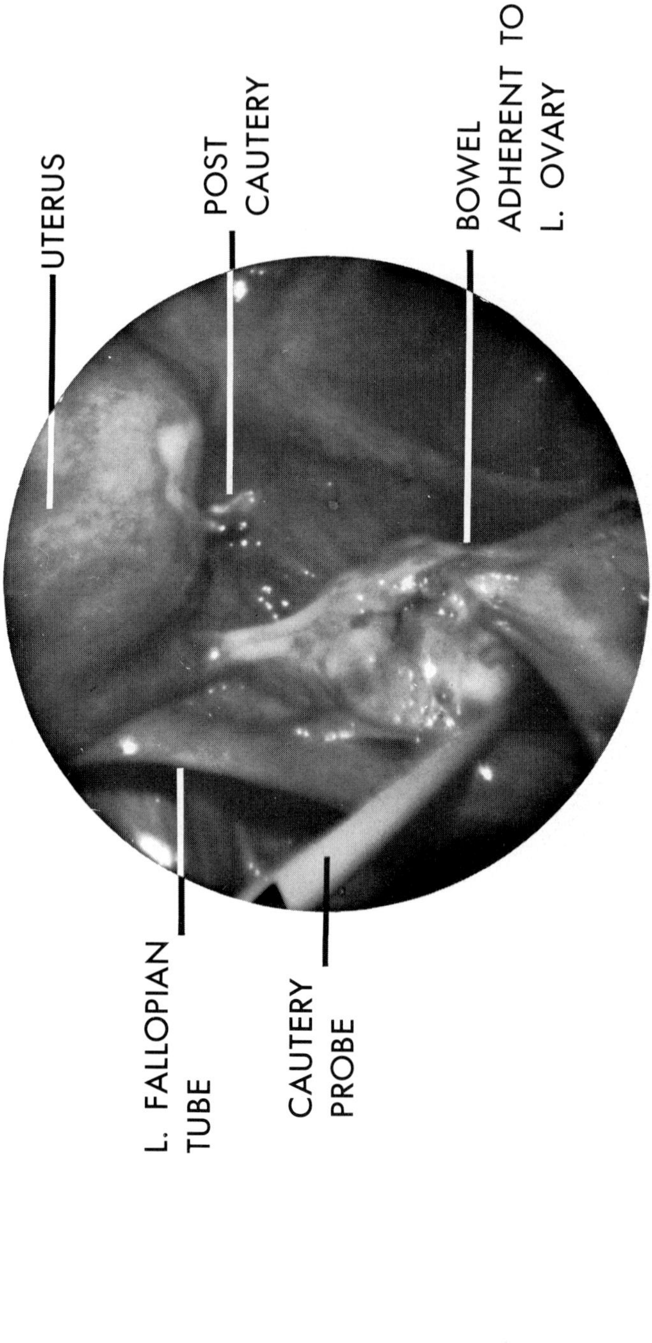


*Figure 17–41.* Laparoscopy. Same patient as in Figure 17–40. Adhesion to uterus severed with Bovie current. It was deemed unwise to separate knuckle of small bowel adherent to the ovary.

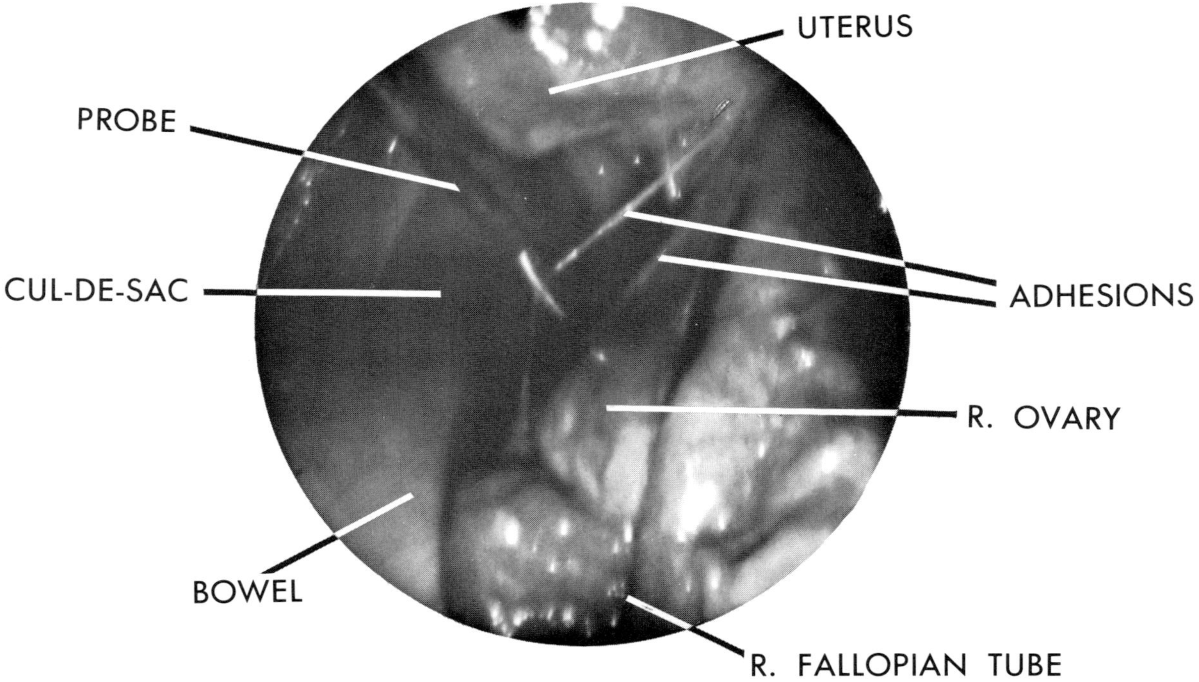


*Figure 17–42.* Laparoscopy. Right adnexa covered with fine adhesions. Cautery probe in position for lysis of adhesions.

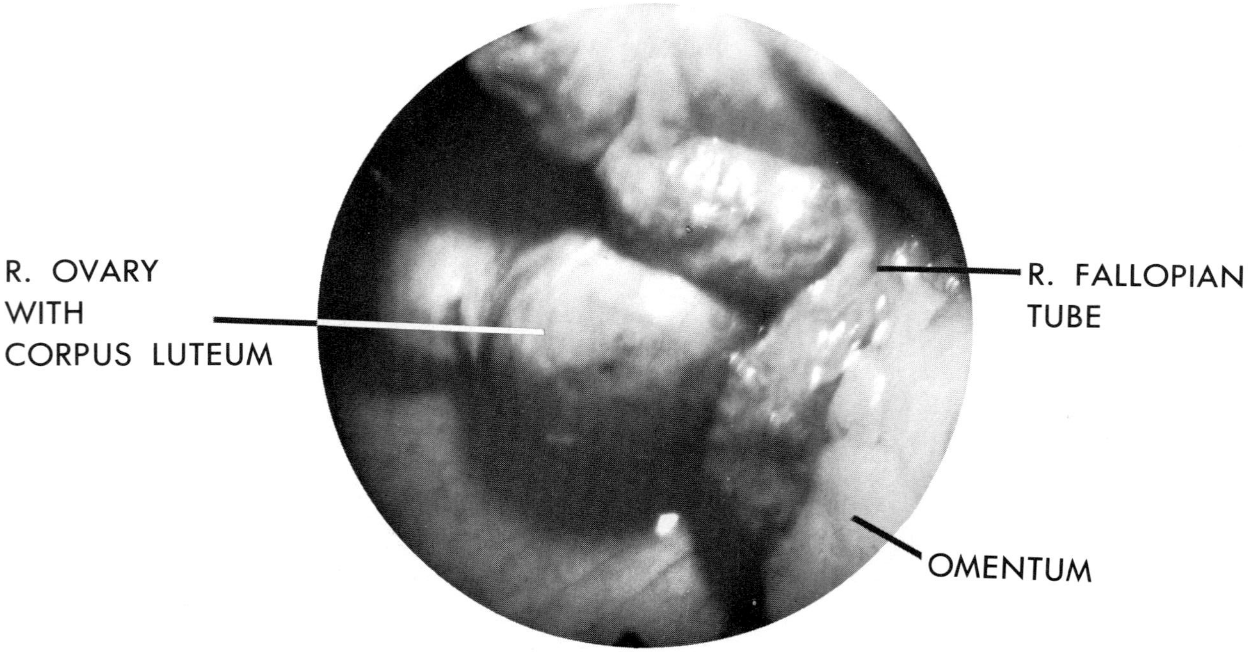


*Figure 17–43.* Laparoscopy. Same patient as in Figure 17–42. Adnexa after lysis of adhesions.

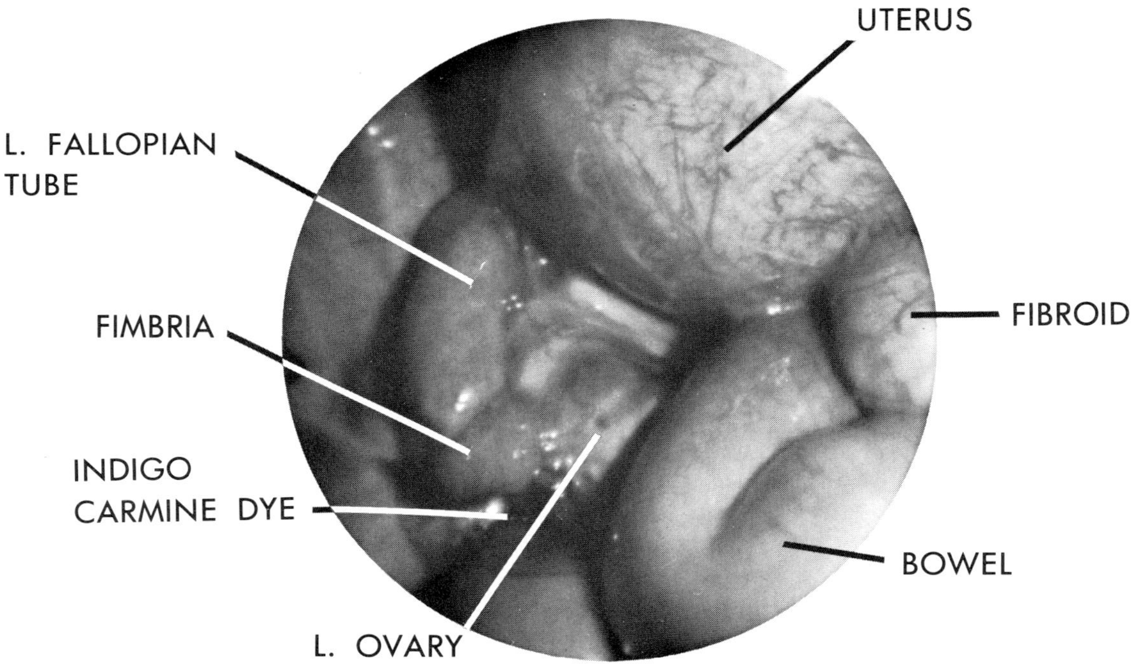


*Figure 17–44.* Laparoscopy. Prior myomectomy and salpingostomy. Note recurrent fibroid, corpus luteum of left ovary, and the shortened, thickened tube with apparently normal fimbria patent to indigo carmine.

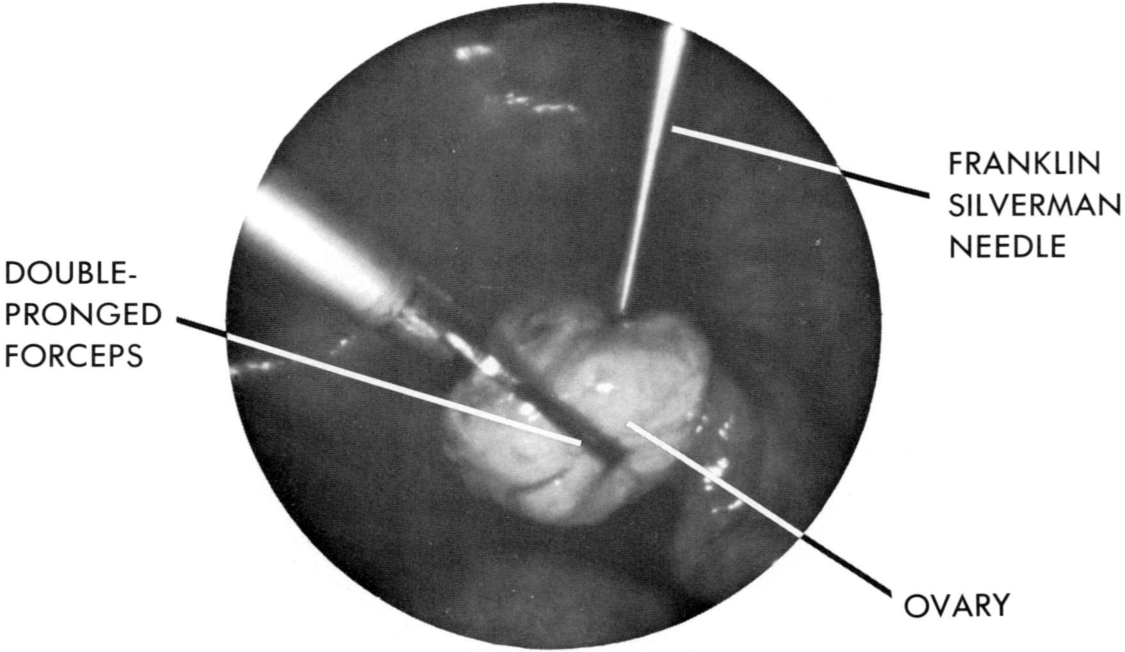


*Figure 17–45.* Laparoscopic demonstration of ovarian biopsy. Ovary is grasped with Palmer or Cohen-Eder biopsy tong so that biopsy needle can penetrate ovary.

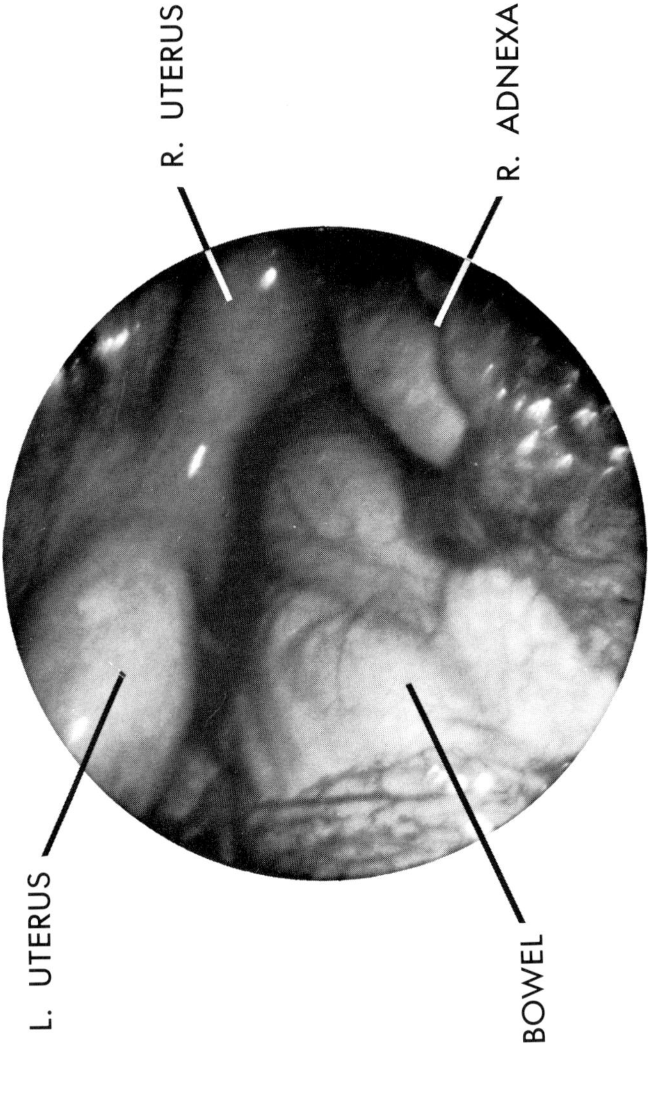


*Figure 17–46.* Laparoscopy. Patient with double uterus and normal right adnexa.

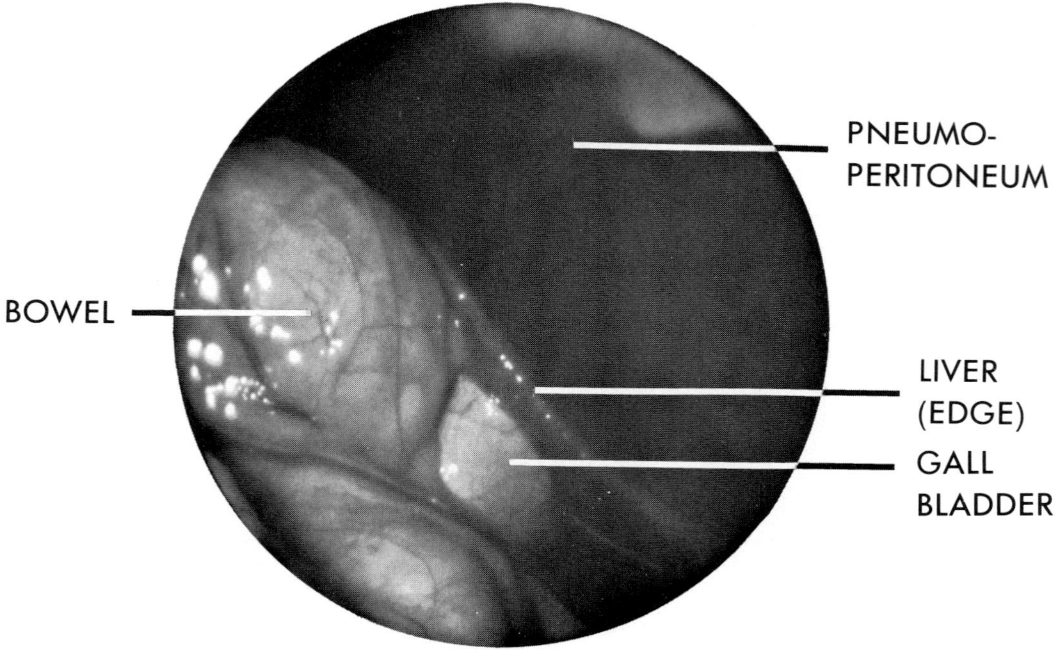


*Figure 17–47.* Upper abdominal laparoscopy demonstrating a normal liver and gallbladder. Note how the pneumoperitoneum separates the liver from the anterior abdominal wall.

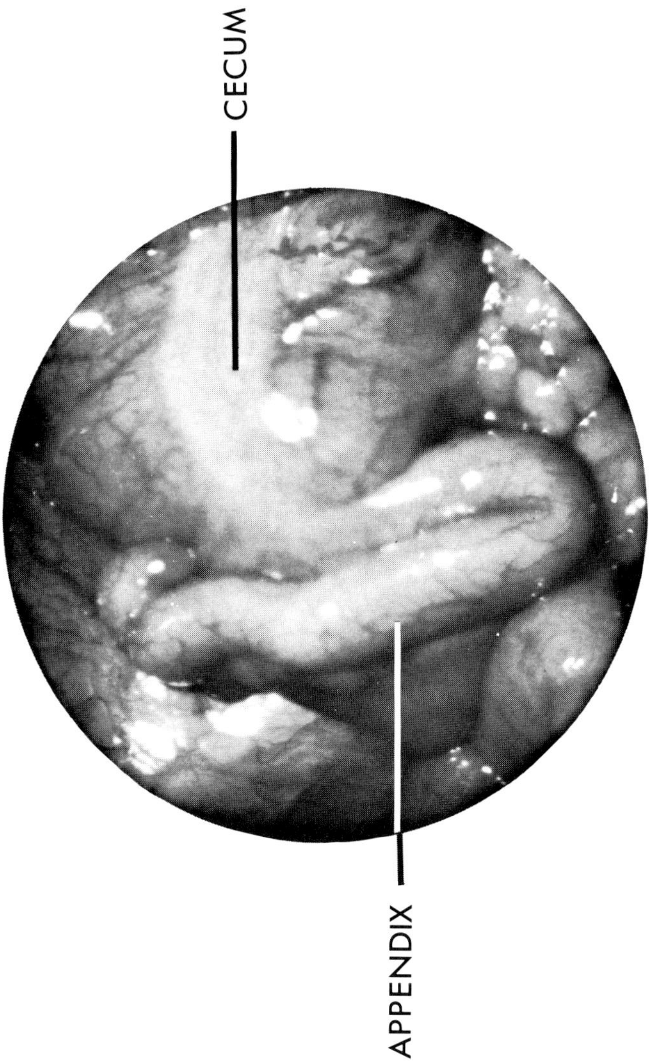


*Figure 17–48.* Laparoscopic demonstration of normal cecum and appendix.

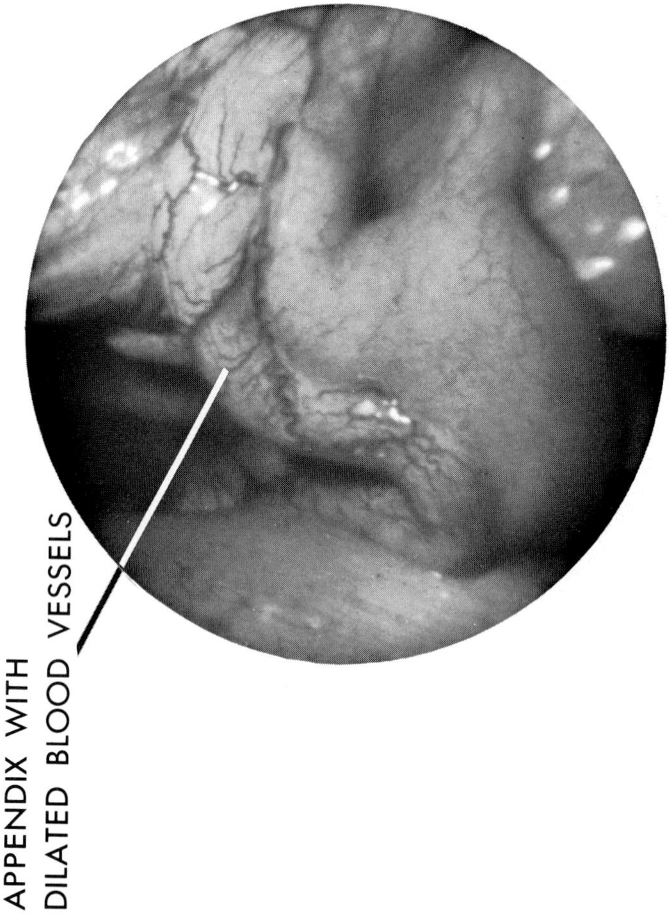


*Figure 17–49.* Acute appendicitis diagnosed via laparoscopy.

# BIBLIOGRAPHY

*BOOKS*

Albano, V., and Cittadini, E. (1962): La Celioscopia in Ginecologia. Denaro, Palermo.

Bailey, H. (1967): Emergency Surgery, Ed. 8. Edited by T. J. McNair, M.D. Williams & Wilkins Co., Baltimore.

Banyai, A. L. (1946): Pneumoperitoneum Treatment. The C. V. Mosby Co., St. Louis.

Benedict, E. B. (1951): Endoscopy. Williams & Wilkins Co., Baltimore.

Decker, A. (1967): Culdoscopy. F. A. Davis Co., Philadelphia.

Frangenheim, H. (1959): Die Laparoskopie und die Culdoskopie in der Gynaekologie. G. Thieme, Stuttgart.

Friedberg, C. K. (1966): Disease of the Heart, Ed. 3. W. B. Saunders Co., Philadelphia.

Kalk, H., and Bruhl, W. (1951): Leitfaden der Laparoskopie und Gastroskopie. G. Thieme, Stuttgart.

Kalk, H., and Wildhirt, E. (1962): Lehrbuch und Atlas der Laparoskopie und Leberpunktion. G. Thieme, Stuttgart.

Korbsch, R. (1927): Lehrbuch und Atlas der Laparoskopie. I. F. Lehmann, Munich.

Palmer, R. (1963): Les Explorations Fonctionelles Gynécologiques. Masson et Cie., Paris.

Stein, A., and Stewart, W. H. (1919): Pneumoperitoneal Roentgen-ray Diagnosis. Southworth Co., Troy, New York.

Steptoe, P. C. (1967): Laparoscopy in Gynaecology. E. & S. Livingston Ltd., Edinburgh and London.

Thoyer-Rozat, J. (1962): La Coelioscopie. Masson et Cie., Paris.

Wildhirt, E. (1964): Bedeutung und Wert der Laparoskopie und Gezielten Leberpunktion. G. Thieme, Stuttgart.

Williams, W. W. (1953): Sterility: The Diagnostic Survey of the Infertile Couple. Walter W. Williams, Springfield, Mass.

Wittman, I. (1966): Peritoneoscopy. Publishing House of the Hungarian Academy of Sciences, Budapest.

*PERIODICALS*

Alexander, G. D., Noe, G. D., and Brown, E. M. (1969): Anesthesia for pelvic laparoscopy. Anesth. Analg. (Paris) *48*:14.

Alvarez, W. C. (1921): Use of $CO_2$ in pneumoperitoneum. Amer. J. Roentgen. *8*:71.

Anderson, E. T. (1937): Peritoneoscopy. Amer. J. Surg. *35*:136.

Balin, H., Wan, L. S., and Israel, S. L. (1966): Recent Advances in Pelvic Endoscopy. Obstet. Gynec. *27*:30.

Beling, C. A. (1939): Experiences in diagnosis with peritoneoscopy and its indications. J. Med. Soc. New Jersey *36*:602.

Beling, C. A. (1941): Selection of cases for peritoneoscopy. Arch. Surg. (Chicago) *42*:872.

Benedict, E. B. (1938): Peritoneoscopy. New Eng. J. Med. *218*:713.

Berenyi, K. J., Sakarya, I., and Snow, J. C. (1966): Innovar nitrous oxide anesthesia in otolaryngology. Laryngoscope *76*:772.

Bernheim, B. M. (1911): Organoscopy: cystoscopy of the abdominal cavity. Ann. Surg. *53*:764.

Clyman, M. J. (1963): A new panculdoscope—diagnostic, photographic, and operative aspects. Obstet. Gynec. *21*:343.
Clyman, M. J. (1968): Operative culdoscopy. Obstet. Gynec. *32*:840.
Cohen, M. R. (1958): Sterility and infertility: medical views. J.A.M.A. *168*:1963.
Cohen, M. R. (1964): Culdoscopy. *In* Williams, W. W.: Sterility: The Diagnostic Survey of the Infertile Couple, Ed. 3. W. W. Williams, Springfield, Mass.
Cohen, M. R. (1966): Stein-Leventhal syndrome: resection versus clomiphene therapy. Fertil. Steril. *17*:765.
Cohen, M. R. (1968*a*): Culdoscopy vs. peritoneoscopy. Obstet. Gynec. *31*:310.
Cohen, M. R. (1968*b*): Ovarian biopsy via peritoneoscopy. J. Reprod. Med. *1*:436.
Cohen, M. R., and Guterman, H. S. (1953): A pelvic photoscope. Obstet. Gynec. *1*:544.
Dasher, W. A., Black, J. P. M., Weiss, W., and Bogen, E. (1954): Air embolism complicating pneumoperitoneum. Amer. Rev. Tuberc. *69*:396.
Decker, A. (1949): Culdoscopy: its diagnostic value in pelvic disease. J.A.M.A. *140*:378.
Decker, A. (1952): Culdoscopy. Amer. J. Obstet. Gynec. *63*:654.
Decker, A., and Cherry, T. (1944): Culdoscopy: a new method in diagnosis of pelvic disease. Amer. J. Surg. *64*:40.
Fear, R. (1968): Laparoscopy: a valuable aid in gynecological diagnosis. Obstet. Gynec. *31*:297.
Fervers, C. (1933): Die Laparoskopie mit dem Cystoskop. Ein Beitrag zur Vereinfachung der Technik und zur Endoskopischen Strangdurchtrennung in der Bauchhöhle, Med. Klin. *29*:1042.
Frangenheim, H. (1957): Vortrag; Sitzung Niederrhein. Westf. Gesell. Gyn. Geburtsh. *131*.
Frangenheim, H. (1958*a*): Vortrag; Sitzung Mittelrhein. Gesell. Gyn. Geburtsh. (Frankfurt).
Frangenheim, H. (1958*b*): Vortrag; Tagung für Medizin. Photographie und Kinematographie.
Frangenheim, H. (1960): Erfahrungen mit der Laparoskopie und der Kuldoskopie in der Gynäkologie. Med. Welt (Berl.) *41*:2152.
Frangenheim, H. (1964*a*): Die Vorteile der Kuldoskopie und der Laparoskopie bei der Diagnose der Extrauteringraviditat. Geburtsh. u. Frauenheilk. *6*:474.
Frangenheim, H. (1964*b*): Die Coelioskopie bei der Sterilitatsuntersuchung. Internat. Symp. Gyn. Celio. (Nov.) 195.
Frangenheim, H. (1965): Technical Errors in Peritoneoscopy. German Med. Monthly *10*:405.
Frangenheim, H. (1968): Vergleichende Untersuchungen Zwischen dem Wert der Pertubation und der Hydrotubation unter Sicht mit dem Coelioskop. Fertil. u. Steril. *10*:190.
Garb, A. E. (1957): A review of tubal sterilization failures. Obstet. Gynec. Survey *12*:291.
Glenn, F. (1953): Cardiac arrest during surgery. Ann. Surg. *137*:920.
Goetze, O. (1918): Die Röntgendiagnostik bei Gasgefullter Bauchhöhle; Eine neue Methode. Münch. Med. Wschr. *65*:1275.
Greenblatt, R. B., Barfield, W. E., Jungck, E. C., and Ray, A. W. (1961): Induction of ovulation with MRL/41. J.A.M.A. *178*:101.
Handley, R. S. (1955): Peritoneoscopy. Postgrad. Med. J. *31*:81.
Handley, R. S., and Nurick, A. W. (1956): Peritoneoscopy; evaluation and report of 136 cases. Brit. Med. J. *2*:1211.
Hartleib, J. (1955): Luftembolie bei der Laparoskopie. Dtsch. Med. Wschr. *80/2*:1532.
Henning, N. (1950): Ein neues Laparoskop. Dtsch. Z. Verdau.-u, Stoffwechselkr. *10*:49.
Henning, N., and Mancke, R. (1933): Die Bedeutung Endoskopischer Methoden fur die Diagnose von Lebererkrangungen. Münch. Med. Wschr. *80*:606.
Heuser, C. (1924): Technic for and findings with roentgenography of ovaries with or without contrast suspension on pneumoperitoneum. Sem. Méd. *2*:1496.
Hope, R. B. (1937): Differential diagnosis of ectopic gestation by peritoneoscopy. Surg. Gynec. Obstet. *64*:229.
Horan, T. N. (1937): Use of the laparoscope. J. Mich. Med. Soc. *36*:634.
Horan, T. N., and Eddy, C. G. (1941): Intra-abdominal photography in color. Surg. Gynec. Obstet. *73*:273.

Hörmann, J. (1955): Mediastinal Emphysem bei der Laparoskopie. Münch. Med. Wschr. *97*:541.
Jacobaeus, H. C. (1910): Ueber die Moglichkeit die Zystoskope bei Untersuchung seroser Höhlung Anzuwenden. Münch. Med. Wschr. *57*:2090.
Jacobeaus, H. C. (1911): Kurze Übersicht über mei Erfahrungen mit der Laparothorakoskopie. Münch. Med. Wschr. *58*:2017.
Jacobaeus, H. C. (1912*a*): Laparo-thorakoskopie. Hygiea (Stockh.) *74*:1070.
Jacobaeus, H. C. (1912*b*): Über Laparo- und Thorakoskopie. Beitr. Klin. Tuberk. *25*:183.
Jernstrom, P. (1951): Air embolism during peritoneoscopy. Amer. J. Clin. Path. *21*:573.
Johnsson, A. (1916): Bidrag till Kannedomen om Laparo-ochtorakoskopi. Finska Läk.-sällsk Handl. *58*:719.
Kalk, H. (1929): Erfahrungen mit der Laparoskopie (Zugleich mit Beschreibung eines neuen Instrumentes). Z. Klin. Med. *111*:303.
Kalk, H. (1935): Laparoskopie. (Die Besichtigung der Bauchhöhle am Lebenden Menschen.) Ges. Krankenh. *5*:97.
Kalk, H., Bruhl, W., and Sieke, E. (1943): Die Gezielte Leberpunktion. Dtsch. Med. Wschr. *69*:693.
Kelling, G. (1902): Über Oesophagoskopie, Gastroskopie und Kölioskopie. Münch. Med. Wschr. *49*:21.
Kelling, G. (1910): Über die Möglichkeit, die Zystoskopie bei Untersuchungen Seroser Höhlungen Anzuwenden. Bemerkung zu dem Artikel von Jacobaeus. Munch. Med. Wschr. *57*:2358.
Kelling, G. (1923): Zur Coelioskopie und Gastroskopie. Arch. Klin. Chir. *126*:226.
Kistner, R. W. (1965*a*): Further observations on the effects of clomiphene citrate in anovulatory females. Amer. J. Obstet. Gynec. *92*:380.
Kistner, R. W. (1965*b*): Induction of ovulation with clomiphene citrate. Obstet. Gynec. Survey *20*:873.
Korbsch, R. (1921): Die Laparoskopie, nach Jacobaeus. Berl. Klin. Wschr. *58*:696.
Korbsch, R. (1922): Technik und Grenzen der Laparoskopie. Münch. Med. Wschr. *69*:426.
Meigs, J. V. (1939): Report of medical progress: gynecology. New Eng. J. Med. *220*:242.
Motschmann, H. (1954): Pneumothorax als Zwischenfall bei der Laparoskopie. Med. Klin. *49*:401.
Nadeau, O. E., and Kampmeier, O. F. (1925): Endoscopy of the abdomen: abdominoscopy. A preliminary study, including a summary of the literature and a description of the technique. Surg. Gynec. Obstet. *41*:259.
Nissen, K. (1954): Laparoskopie. Schweiz. Med. Wschr. *84*:293.
Nordentoeft, S. (1912): Über Endoskopie Geschlossener Cavitaten mittels eines Trokar-Endoskops. Verh. Dtsch. Ges. Chir. *41*:78.
Orndoff, B. H. (1920): The peritoneoscope in diagnosis of diseases of the abdomen. J. Radiol. *1*:307.
Ott, D. O. (1901): Ventroscopic illumination of the abdominal cavity in pregnancy. Z. Akus i Zhensk. Bolez. *15*:7.
Ott, D. O. (1902): Die Beleuchtung der Bauchhöhle (Ventroskopie) als Methode bei Vaginaler Coeliotomie. Abl. Gynäk. *231*:817.
Palmer, R. (1947): Coelioscopie par la vois transvaginale. C. R. Soc. Franç. Gynéc. *17*:229.
Palmer, R. (1948): La Coelioscopie. Brux.-méd. *28*:305.
Palmer, R. (1954): La Coelioscopie gynécologique, ses possibilités et ses indications actuelles. Sem. Hôp. Paris *30*:4441.
Palmer, R. (1959*a*): Celioscopy in the diagnosis of refractory pelvic pain. Rev. Prat. (Paris) *9*:2375.
Palmer, R. (1959*b*): Celioscopy in amenorrhea. Gaz. Méd. Fr. *66*:1153.
Palmer, R. (1960*a*): What can be expected at the present time from celioscopy in gynecology. Acta Gynaec. Obstet. Hisp.-lusit. 9:19.
Palmer, R. (1960*b*): Progrès Récents et indications actuelles de la coelioscopie abdominale en gynécologie (avec présentation de film). Mém. Acad. Chir. *86*:659.
Peterson, R. (1921): Pneumoperitoneum and roentgenology as aids to more accurate obstetric and gynecologic diagnosis. Amer. J. Obstet. Gynec. *2*:349.

Power, F. H., and Barnes, A. C. (1941): Sterilization by means of peritoneoscopic tubal fulguration. Amer. J. Obstet. Gynec. *41*:1038.
Renon, L. (1913*a*): Valeur de la Laparoscopie. Presse Méd. *21*:700.
Renon, L. (1913*b*): Technique et indications de la laparoscopie (présentation d'instrument). Bull. Soc. Méd. Hôp. Paris *35*:510.
Renon, L. (1913*c*): Technique et indications de la laparoscopie. Rev. Gén. Clin. et Thér. *27*:148.
Renon, L. (1914): La valeur de la laparoscopie. Internat. Congr. Med. London (1913), Sect. VI, *2*:571.
Riegel, R. (1952): Pneumothorax nach Diagnostischem Pneumoperitoneum bei Laparoskopie. Beitr. Klin. Tuberk. *107*:467.
Roccavilla, A. (1914): L'endoscopia delle grandi cavità siercse mediante un movo apparecchio ad illuminazione diretta. Rif. Med. *30*:991.
Roccavilla, A. (1920): Laparoscopia e pneumoradiologie abdominale. Radiol. Med. (Torino) *7*:411.
Rosenbaum, F. J. (1954): Die Cholangiographie; Ihre Technik und Diagnostische Bedeutung. Münch. Med. Wschr. *96*:573.
Rosenbaum, F. J. (1955): Die Laparoskopische. Klin. Wschr. *33*:39.
Rosenbaum, F. J. (1958): Gefahren und Kontraindikationen der Laparoskopie, Besonders der Leber- und Milzpunktion. Dtsch. Med. Wschr. *83*:222.
Rosenthal, G. (1913): Le laparothoracoscope de Jacobaeus. Bull. Gén. Thér. (Paris) *165*:802.
Rosner, K. (1955): Mediastinalemphysema bei Laparoskopie. Münch. Med. Wschr. *97*:1367.
Roy, S., Greenblatt, R. B., Mahesh, V. B., and Jungck, E. C. (1963): Clomiphene citrate: further observations on its use in induction of ovulation in the human and on its mode of action. Fertil. Steril. *14*:540.
Royer, M. (1945): Laparoscopia o peritoneoscopia; su estado actual. Prens. Méd. Argent. *32*:1255.
Ruddock, J. C. (1934): Peritoneoscopy. West. J. Surg. *42*:392.
Ruddock, J. C. (1937): Peritoneoscopy. Surg. Gynec. Obstet. *65*:623.
Ruddock, J. C. (1939): Peritoneoscopy. Sth. Surg. *8*:113.
Ruddock, J. C. (1949): Application and evaluation of peritoneoscopy. Calif. Med. *71*:110.
Ruddock, J. C. (1957): Peritoneoscopy; a critical clinical review. Surg. Clin. N. Amer. *37*:1249.
Schmidt, A. (1914): Laparoskopie und Thorakoskopie nach Jacobaeus. Münch. Med. Wschr. *61*:1882.
Shackelford, R. T. (1941): Peritoneoscopy. Surgery *10*:742.
Siegler, A. M., and Berenyi, K. J. (1969): Laparoscopy in gynecology. Obstet. Gynec. *34*:572.
Stein, A. (1919): Oxygen peritoneal inflation before x-ray. Ann. Surg. *70*:95.
Stein, A., and Stewart, W. H. (1919): Roentgen-ray study of abdominal organs following oxygen inflation of peritoneal cavity. Amer. J. Roentgen. *6*:533.
Stein, I. F. (1937): Why pneumoperitoneum? Radiology *28*:391.
Stein, I. F. (1943): Gynecography: X-ray diagnosis in gynecology. Surg. Clin. N. Amer. *23*:165.
Stein, I. F. (1964): Duration of fertility following ovarian wedge resection: Stein-Leventhal syndrome. West. J. Surg. *72*:237.
Stein, I. F., and Arens, R. A. (1930): Visualization of the pelvic viscera. Radiology *15*:85.
Stein, I. F., and Leventhal, M. L. (1935): Amenorrhea associated with bilateral polycystic ovaries. Amer. J. Obstet. Gynec. *29*:181.
Stein, I. F., Cohen, M. R., and Elson, R. (1949): Results of bilateral ovarian wedge resection in 47 cases of sterility. Amer. J. Obstet. Gynec. *58*:267.
Steinberg, U. (1956): Komplikationen bei der Laparoskopie I. Beobachtungen bei Anlegung des Pneumoperitoneums. Z. Ges. Inn. Med. *11*:557.
Steiner, O. P. (1924*a*): Abdominoskopie. Schweiz. Med. Wschr. *54*:84.
Steiner, O. P. (1924*b*): Abdominoscopy. Surg. Gynec. Obstet. *38*:266.
Stephenson, H. E., Jr., Reid, L. C., and Hinton, J. W. (1953): Some common denominators in 1200 cases of cardiac arrest. Ann. Surg. *137*:731.

Steptoe, P. C. (1967): A new method of tubal sterilization. Proceedings of the Fifth World Congress on Fertility and Sterility (Stockholm) *133*:1183.

Steptoe, P. C. (1969): Personal communication.

Stewart, W. N., and Stein, I. F. (1919): X-ray study of the abdominal organs following oxygen inflation of the peritoneal cavity. Amer. J. Roentgenol. *6*:533.

Stiefel, G. E. (1961): Über die Gefahren, Kontraindikationen und Indikationen der Laparoskopie, der Gesielten und Blinden Leberbiopsie. Schweiz. Med. Wschr. *4*:97.

Strauss, H. A., and Cohen, M. R. (1955): Gynecography simplified. Amer. J. Obstet. Gynec. *70*:572.

Taylor, M. B. (1969): Instrument and method: headpiece clamp for the peritoneoscope. Obstet. Gynec. *33*:124.

Tedesko, F. (1912): Über Endoskopie des Abdomens und des Thorax. Mitt. Gesch. Inn. Med. Kinderh. in Wien *12*:323.

Towbin, M. (1951): Mediastinal emphysema occurring during therapeutic pneumoperitoneum. Ann. Intern. Med. *35*:555.

Turner, H. H. (1938): A syndrome of infantilism, congenital webbed neck and cubitus valgus. Endocrinology *23*:566.

Vilardell, F., Seres, I., and Marti-Vicente, A. (1968): Complications of peritoneoscopy: A survey of 1,455 examinations. Gastro. Endoscop. *14*:178.

Walker, R. M., and Playfair, P. L. (1942): Peritoneoscopy: report based on 125 cases. Lancet *1*:159.

Walker, R. M., Cooke, A. M., and Playfair, P. L. (1943): Peritoneoscopy. Proc. Roy. Soc. Med. *36*:445.

Wenderoth, H. (1954): Nil Nocere!: Mediastinalemphysema bei Laparoskopie. Münch. Med. Wschr. *96*:1369.

West, J. P. (1954): Cardiac arrest during anesthesia and surgery. Ann. Surg. *140*:623.

Wildhirt, K. (1955): Die Medicamentose Behandlung der Diffusen Leberparenchymerkrankungen. Med. Klin. *29*:980.

Wildhirt, K. (1956): Mediastinalemphysem bei Laparoskopie und zur Luftembolie bei Laparoskopie. Münch. Med. Wschr. *98*:58.

Wittman, I., Aszodi, Z., and Papp, L. (1964): Festékoldatok Újabb Alkalmazása a Diagnosztikában. I. Chromolaparoskópia. (Recent use of stains in diagnostics. I. Chromoperitoneoscopy). Orv. Hetil. *105*(10):447.

Yung, P. (1923): Radiographie des organes de petit bassin de la femme après pneumoperitoine. Gynec. et Obstet. *8*:329.

Zollikofer, R. (1924): Zur Laparoskopie. Schweiz. Med. Wschr. *54*:264.

# Index

Note: Page numbers in *italics* refer to illustrations; (t) refers to tables.